CHOICES

Planning the Rest of Your Life

Leslie Baldwin

Copyright © 2003 by Leslie Baldwin.

Library of Congress Number: 2003097770
ISBN :   Hardcover   1-4134-3278-6
         Softcover   1-4134-3277-8

All rights reserved. No part of this book may be reproduced or transmitted in any form or by any means, electronic or mechanical, including photocopying, recording, or by any information storage and retrieval system, without permission in writing from the copyright owner.

This book was printed in the United States of America.

To order additional copies of this book, contact:
Xlibris Corporation
1-888-795-4274
www.Xlibris.com
Orders@Xlibris.com
20352

CONTENTS

INTRODUCTION 11

ACKNOWLEDGEMENTS 15

CHAPTER ONE—Aging Is All About Living 17
    Oh No! Not Another "How To" Book! 17
    Aging Happens. Staying Healthy Takes Work 19
    Thrive—Don't Just Survive 20
    When you Think About Aging—
        Think Great Wine 20
    Who Me? I'll Never Grow Old! 23
    You Have to Know and Like Yourself
        to Move Successfully Into and Through any
        New Phase of Your Life. 27
    The Secret To Problem Solving is Finding
        the Information and Services We Need 27
    Thinking About the Finale 30

CHAPTER TWO—Retirement Planning
    Starts Sooner Than We Think 32
    The Care and Feeding of the Retired Business, Military,
        Medical, Corporate, and/or
        Compulsive Workaholic Person 33
    For the Partner, Contemplating Retirement
        May Not be So Simple 34
    LOVE is a Four Letter Word 39
    Know What Questions to Ask About Retirement 40

CHAPTER THREE—A Healthy Attitude May be the Best Medicine 43
   A Nutritionist Should be Your New Best Friend 45
   A Geriatric Specialist Can Save Your Life 46
   Getting in the Mood 47
   Staying Healthy
      By Learning About The Changing Body 50
   Some Examples of What our Bodies
      are Trying to Tell Us 51
   So Many New Theories, Therapies
      and Puzzles to Sift Through 56
   Eating Well Can Help Keep us Well 57
   Many of us Eat Too Much 58
   Reading the Labels—"Lite"
      is Not Necessarily Low Fat or Low Calorie 60
   Evaluate New Studies on Food
      With a Healthy Skepticism 64
   Being Overweight Can Bring
      Chronic Health Problems at Any Age 65
   Exercise—The Best Anti-Aging Medicine There is 66
   Why Does It Feel So Bad
      When I Enjoyed Eating it so Much? 70
   Medicine Doesn't Always Make us Well 76
   Alcohol. How's a Body to Know? 84
   Getting a Good Night's Sleep Can be a Challenge 86
   Risk Free Sneezing—
      How To Hold Incontinence at Bay 91

CHAPTER FOUR—When Staying Healthy Doesn't Work 94
   Battling Chronic and Serious Illness 95
   The Communication Age is Here.
      But Use it Wisely 98
   Becoming an Active Member of the Team 103
   What Everyone Should Know
      About Heart Disease 109

Would I Recognize a Stroke or
   Brain Attack if I were Having One? 111
Guess what . . . Men Get Breast Cancer Too! 113
What Every Man and Woman Should Know About
   Prostate Cancer 115
Alternative or Complimentary Medicine
   and Integrative Therapies...................................... 117
If The Doctor Recommends Surgery 124
How to be an Effective Medical Advocate 129
Decoding, Demystifying
   and Surviving the Medical Bills 135
A Medical Profile Could Save Your Life
   in an Emergency 138

CHAPTER FIVE—Recovery, Healing and Caregiving 139
   Concentrating on Healing and Recovery
      After a Hospital Stay 140
   Caring for Someone Else . . .
      a Cram Course in Planning for Oneself............. 141
   Negotiating a Minefield—
      Dealing with Ghosts of Relationships Past......... 149
   When Some Nursing Care is Necessary 150
   Levels of Care Available 152
   Types of Private Home Health/Nursing Care 153
   Finding the Best Caregiver 155
   Caring for Someone From a Long Way Away 167
   Searching for a Nursing Home
      is a Complicated Process 169
   We Should Never Accept Abuse
      for Ourselves or for Anyone Else........................ 172
   Hospice is Another Word for
      End of Life Caring 175

CHAPTER SIX—Understanding Depression
   and Memory Loss 177
   Depression is No Longer a "Hidden" Illness 178

Memory Doesn't Have To Be
  The First Thing To Go 188
Dementia Syndrome 192
Pseudodementia 193
Multi-Infarct Dementia 195
Alzheimer's Disease, (AD) 195
Being a Caregiver For the AD Patient 203
Medicare Rules on Early Treatment for AD 205

**CHAPTER SEVEN—Turning Worry About The Future
  Into A Positive Exercise** 207
Bringing Adult Children Into the Equation 207
A Sound Partnership Calls for Full Disclosure 209
Preparing for the Unthinkable—
  Becoming Suddenly Single 211
Do Your Heirs a Favor.
  Create a Personal Information File 212
Don't Become a Victim of Identity Theft 214
If Everything I Had Was Lost Today,
  Would I Know What was Gone? 217
An Elder Law Service Could Help
  with Planning for the Future 219
Estate Planning, Wills, Trusts
  and Health Care Decisions 220
Financial Planning 221
Medical and Long Term Health Care Planning 224
Planning for Incapacity 229
Update Documents Periodically 234

**CHAPTER EIGHT—Maintaining a Certain Style
  of Living** 235
Encourage Trusting Relationships—
  Networking Before You Need it 237
Designing an Exit Strategy 241
Senior Citizen Apartment Complexes and/or
  Retirement Communities 246

Home-share or the Nontraditional Home Setting 247
Assisted Living Facilities 248
Continuing or Lifetime Care Communities 249
Moving in With the Children 253
Face the Music—Moving Day
    is Just Around the Corner 255
It's Never Too Late to Learn Something New 261
Being a Grandparent.
    The Best Deal in the World 264
Staying in the Driver's Seat as Long as Possible 272
Shake the Dust From Your Traveling Shoes 279
Turning Disabilities Into Possibilities 283
Making Life Easier Can Be Stylish and Fun 287
Cleaning up our Act 288

CHAPTER NINE—Planning the Curtain Call
Before the Finale **290**
Putting Everything in One Place 292
Where There's a Will, There Should Be a Way 292
Being an Executor. It's Not Always an Honor 297
The Funeral—Having it Your Way 299
The Obituary—
    How I Would Like to Be Remembered 301
Live On and On as an Organ Donor 303
Grieving is a Survival Skill 304
Leaving a Legacy 306
Bringing the Family Out of the Closet 309
Finding a Place for Professional Papers
    and Pictures 311
Storing, Preserving and Protecting our Treasures 312
Clearing Out a Family Home
    Can be an Emotional Roller Coaster 314
Strategies for Sharing the Memories
    and the Valuables 316
And so the Finale is a Beginning 320

This book is dedicated to those spirited men and women
Who have shown us the way to live with wisdom and grace.

And to Jack, Dorothy and Sam,
Charlie and Mo, Michael and Stuart
Whose wife, mother, mother-in-law and grandmother
I am proud to be.

INTRODUCTION

One phone call 13 years ago set me on the path to writing this book. My 84-year-old mother asked me to take her to the doctor where she learned that she had pancreatic cancer and with surgery could count on only four months to live. In the subsequent six months I learned a lot about helping a loved one survive a hospital stay and setting up a system of home health care. We appreciated end of life care for my mother dispensed by Hospice as they helped her and us in her last moments. During her illness and after her death we became wiser to the fact that health care providers' skills and commitment vary widely and also that one needs to be more knowledgeable about procedure in order to be able to wade through the legal and bureaucratic requirements of death. Settling the estate and preparing the house for sale made me vow never to allow myself to leave so many issues unresolved for our children to go through after we are gone.

Since then, my husband and I have assisted several relatives and friends who have reached "very old" status without a clear picture of how they would be able to manage increased incapacity in a very changed world. The common denominators for most of these people, who happened to be women were, a determination to be independent, a will of iron and the embrace of a plan of inaction called denial. This book is the result of my promise to myself that we would learn how to plan ahead long before the vagaries of chance or the limits of aging bring about changes in our lifestyle; that I would make myself aware of ways to stay healthy and, when circumstances called for it, to try to restore health by being actively involved in decisions made about my own treatment and care if I became ill.

I have always believed that nutrition holds the key to good health. This is why I have drawn so extensively on the knowledge and wisdom of my friend Charlotte Gollobin, a certified nutritionist. She knows about the changes that occur to our bodies in aging, and how those changes affect the assimilation of food, medicines and supplements; but, more importantly, she never stops searching and learning. If we are to make wise choices for ourselves, we too need this knowledge. Charlotte has consistently been a step ahead of many of the theories, which have become widely accepted in the last 15 years. But she has also stressed the importance of viewing those theories with common sense and a clear understanding of how they might affect each individual differently.

I found there was a lot of information in the public sector for the caregivers of elderly parents but precious little for people like me who wanted to strategize a holistic approach to physical, emotional and financial health as I moved from middle to old age and possibly into very old age. I want to move from trusting in luck to acknowledging that fate can change the balance of life in a split second no matter what my age. As friends heard of my project, I became a source of information in their quest to solve problems for their elderly parents and found that giving them the resources they needed was an opening to convince them that they should be concerned about their own future as well.

My experience working with Navy families taught me how to resolve issues associated with a mobile lifestyle. Frequent moves, having to create a place for ourselves in each new community while helping others do the same, and the raising of a family with one parent gone a lot of the time taught me how to find the help I needed and learn to be independent. Interviews conducted and anecdotes related illustrate how the information I have collected can work for all of us. But it also shows how unique each one of us is and that one model solution does not fit all.

I have been asked for whom this book is written. The answer is difficult to pin down. It is to address situations faced as the adult child of our parents and the aging parent of our children. I am looking for a way to move into my own future with confidence thus this book is an attempt to share what I have learned. It is to make others aware of the pitfalls of not planning for the future, and to show them how to find the resources available to help them and their parents. It is for the "very old" person who has mobility needs. It is also for the person of any age who hasn't seen to documents like a Living Will, entrusted someone with a Durable Health Care Power of Attorney or decided who to ask to be a medical advocate if he or she should have to be admitted to a hospital.

If each of us has done our homework, our children will be reassured that not only do we wish to remain in control of our own destiny as long as we are able, but also that we are flexible enough to make the hard decisions to stay in at least partial control as long as possible. Having the confidence to welcome each new stage of life with grace and acceptance takes training and the skill of problem solving. This book is filled with information that any of us can access from the public sector in magazines, newspapers, the Internet and books on these issues. It covers such a wide range of subjects that I hope you will use the resources to study the ones that interest you in more depth. What I hope you will discover is how to look for what you want, how to let a discontinued phone number or a vanished Web site be a link to finding information another way. I have had interviews with experts in differing fields and those who are living the experience of growing older who shared their thoughts with generosity. It is in the selection of the subjects I have chosen to cover that I express my hope for the future, my joy in sharing the lessons I have learned and my undying gratitude to the friends who have helped me complete this book.

And last but not least, I want you to understand that the strategies, resources, advice and counsel found in *Choices, Planning the Rest of Your Life* can in no way take the place of a consultation with your own doctor or other experts in each field discussed.

ACKNOWLEDGEMENTS

There are so many people who have helped me over the years to write and complete this book that I could not possibly name them all. I list the following names, not in order of the contribution they have made to the project, but alphabetically, because each one, in his or her own way, gave exactly the support needed at just the right moment.

Mo Baldwin, although busy with her own projects, helped me format the book, a task I could not have done by myself. Summerfield Baldwin brought me up to speed on the legal instruments needed for estate and medical purposes. Lisa Block shared with me her sensitive and wise advice on recovery for the very ill person. Ned Campbell verified many of the medical references I made and encouraged me in this project. Jim Connolly, one of those charming van line representatives showed me what a really good moving company can do and then helped me write about it. Rebecca Crowell was the person who started this project with me many years ago and taught me how to research the subjects I wished to cover. Robert Fuller was also one of the first people to encourage and support the project when he was entirely too busy to give me so much time and has continued to do so. Renee Glaser read the draft early on and challenged me to do better. Georgia Gosnell was a thoughtful reader who gave me encouragement and goaded me to finish the project. Jane Harder was one of those persons I interviewed who gave me insight into the rich diversity of personality and independence of the individual. Mary Supplee has been an inspiration and role model since long before I started to do this project and it was her beautiful, honest vision of life that has given the book its theme. Tom Hobbins, an expert on sleep disorders, shared his skills and knowledge generously. Randolph King was one of my early readers and, through some well-chosen pointers, kept me on track. Riley and Annette Mixson shared in intimate detail her successful battle with cancer and told how best to be an advocate for someone who is very ill. Jacqueline Quillen has been my cheerleader, sometime editor, draft reader, inspiration, and good friend. Bob Rich was a reader who came up with valuable insurance information. Audrey Riker, a classmate I haven't seen for a very long time, shared thoughts on the pleasures of children and life lived for others. Harriet Sheehy has been my inspiration, my friend, a never failing well of wisdom and has helped me from the very beginning with advice and counsel through every version of the book. Pat Stearn was the best editor I could have had with her generous comments and insistence on good grammar. Cynthia Steele brought knowledge and compassion to my understanding of Alzheimer's Disease. Susan Xanders reviewed a draft of the book and helped me do a better job on residence options for the elderly.

It is with profound gratitude that I thank them all for their manifold and generous contributions.

CHAPTER ONE

AGING IS ALL ABOUT LIVING

Oh No! Not Another "How To" Book!

During the 90's career patterns changed so dramatically that retirement for some Internet entrepreneurs came as early as 35, or as late as 75 for those who were reluctant to give up working. Although the "go-go" economy that encouraged such activity is now just a memory, the fact remains that planning for retirement and beyond should be more than daydreaming; it should be an ongoing process starting on the first day of work, continuing through each promotion or change of career and into retirement itself.

Not only are Americans living longer, they have access to more information, are educated better about health issues than ever before and, since fitness has become a part of many more lives, are becoming proactive about staying healthy. The numbers show that we could live well past the day once thought of as the moment to retire. We may feel at the top of our game now, but resources, sufficient for immediate needs, must also be available for a time when age and circumstances could make it physically or mentally impossible to complete tasks presently taken for granted, like paying bills and driving to the store. Trying to prepare for what the future brings is to indulge in a game of weighing chance and risk, but not to do so is an even greater gamble. It is easy to postpone thinking about possible trouble spots along the way when things are going well, but past history proves life can change in the blink of an eye.

The impact of chronic and debilitating disease in later life is well documented, particularly by those who have been through it with elderly relatives, but no one can guarantee that those of us who are in middle age now won't become a victim of either one long before "old age." When thinking of our parents or elderly relatives, we may see that they are active and in total control of their daily lives at the moment but the possibility exists that they could, in the not too distant future, need help in ways they never imagined or prepared for, as might you and I.

No "how to" book can solve every challenge encountered as a caregiver, supply the energy to pursue one more lead or the perseverance to come to a decision when emotions cloud the issues. But this book may stimulate the reader to find new ways to approach old problems difficult to solve before. It could teach us how to ask the right questions and back them up with resources when we require assistance ourselves. It could make us understand that we need skill and persistence to get the help we deserve from agencies established to provide that assistance. No one can tell us what we will experience when we find ourselves concerned with the health and welfare of an aging parent while we are bringing up our own children, but a book like this one can help us focus our efforts and provide resources to use our time most effectively.

Even more important, it should make us understand how important it is to think through what we need to do for ourselves to stay independent and productive as long as we can while being realistic about the possibility of problems, which could develop as we age.

Aging Happens. Staying Healthy Takes Work

The law of averages says that we can live to a ripe old age. From the Website of the American Academy of Anti-aging Medicine I found some interesting statistics from the UN. By 2050 seniors will outnumber children for the first time in history and represent the world's fastest growing population segment. There are possibly going to be 3.2 million people 100 or older by that same time. This tells me that we have a real stake in learning to live a healthy lifestyle so that we can enjoy most of those years free from chronic disease usually associated with the aging process. Researchers in the area of anti-aging medicine say that a large percentage of all illness in the elderly is due to the degenerative process of aging hastened by factors such as exposure to pollution, lack of exercise and poor lifestyle choices. They suggest that an emphasis on prevention by using such tools as tests for early detection of disease and attention to fitness can hold off and reverse many of the conditions restricting quality of life for older people. Cholesterol testing and drugs to control it, mammograms, nutritional supplements, exercise, as disease preventive, and research on gene engineering are examples of such anti-aging potential. Modern medicine has given us the tools to improve the odds of staying healthy and active, now we have to take advantage of what they have given us by becoming proactive in managing our own health care.

RESOURCE

The American Academy of Anti-Aging Medicine has a non-profit, public service website with an interesting format for giving one a lot of information on the whole subject of what can be done to find optimum health in terms of diet, lifestyle, medical breakthroughs, prevention, etc. There is also information on individual health challenges in an easy to access format.

www.WorldHealth.net

Thrive—Don't Just Survive

If prolonging a healthy and vigorous life is our goal, proper diet, exercise and attention to yearly screening tests are already a part of our life. But to take full advantage of the wonders of medical science, we have to learn how to be proactive in our search for good medical care and then make it responsive to our particular needs.

The first step in this process is to get into a frame of mind that will encourage the enthusiasm and energy it takes to make it all come true. Birthdays needn't herald a process that moves us away from happiness and into increasingly limited enjoyment. They can be a celebration of where we have been in our lives and an acknowledgement that we foresee a future full of interesting choices. It is now popular wisdom that as the years progress the more optimistic, contented, involved and interested we are, the more successfully we will age.

And last, but not least, exercise your sense of humor. The more you use it the better you can face the nicks and burns that life sometimes puts in your path.

Resource

In this collection of verse welcoming increasing age, there is a section for those of us with adult children and aging parents I found to be particularly comforting.
Too Wise to Want to Be Young Again: A Witty View of How to Stop Counting the Years and Start Living Them
Natasha Josefowitz—Blue Mountain Press—Boulder, Colorado—
ISBN 0-88396-422-8

When you Think About Aging— Think Great Wine

Obviously, thinking about aging is not a joyous event, so it makes more sense and is far more important to think about living. If that doesn't work for you think of yourself as a truly great wine;

a product of careful selection of ingredients, nurtured throughout its youth and middle age by soaking up influences from its environment, aging at its own pace and ready to dazzle at a mature age. Limits to healthy functioning have a great deal to do with genetic factors, financial resources, life experiences, and luck but most important, how we view our own aging. Attitude will help define what elderly means and if there is a time when we consider ourselves old, we may find that we do so with pride. A friend of ours in her 90s is energetic, involved and active, yet her younger sister was an invalid for eight years before her death due to progressive illness. Both had the same genetic background but other environmental, personality and health factors changed the equation. Our friend has been determined to ignore limits imposed by physical discomfort and to remain in control of her life at all costs.

Dr. John Rowe and Robert L. Kahn, in their book *Successful Aging* say that genetic factors account for only 30% of the changes in physical aspects of aging and 50% of changes in mental acuity. It is becoming clearer that we have a lot more control over the health we will enjoy in later life than perhaps we had previously thought. It is impossible to predict what the future holds for any of us, but there are many things we can do to help adjust to changing needs of both mind and body and strengthen out resiliency no matter what chronological age we have reached. There is nothing mysterious about the process. Ignore it and hope for the best or welcome it with understanding and *make* it the best. It helps to understand that growing and aging are what we do from the moment we are born. As with a great bottle of wine, aging is what pulls knowledge, experience and wisdom together and makes us memorable.

Resource

I enjoyed reading this and found it very illuminating.
    Successful Aging
    By Dr. John Rowe and Robert L. Kahn—Delacourt Press—
    1999—ISBN 0-440-50863-0
If any man can be talked into reading about his own aging process, this is the

book to get. If that's not an option, wives can try reading it themselves to get some insight into the male process of aging. Very enlightening.

Understanding Men's Passages Discovering the New Map of Men's Lives—
By Gail Sheehy—Random House—1998—ISBN 0-679-45273-7

The Hard Work is Now
When We Can't Imagine Needing Help

Planning for living is not an exercise in pessimism; it is an attempt to be prepared if things go wrong and to make choices for ourselves rather than trusting to luck. It is possible to strike a balance between living peacefully in the present and preparing for the worst in the future. Divorce, death of a spouse, financial reverses or the loss of a job, retirement, a catastrophic or increasingly debilitating chronic illness qualify as life-changing events which should encourage rethinking a course for the future. When things go "bad wrong," they can go from a manageable situation to an all-consuming struggle in a matter of days or hours. Those of us who have been part of such a struggle with elderly relatives have seen this.

How we react to change as we get older and the flexibility we show in moving away from long held patterns when necessary can be seen as a direct result of adjusting to new opportunities as we go along rather than feeling we are giving up freedoms. If we take measured steps consistent with an overall, well thought out plan we will have gone a long way toward easing a feeling of helplessness when things don't go well.

Resource

I found this book very readable and written by someone who has wide experience with "aging" people. It is great for those who dread growing older.

GROWING OLDER AND WISER Coping with Expectations, Challenges, and Change in the Later Years
By Nathan Billig, M.D.—Lexington Books—1993—*ISBN: 0-669-27678-2*

Who Me? I'll Never Grow Old!

From the information I have been able to gather about Baby Boomers, it appears as though they believe they will never age. That is, they feel that retirement is simply a career change and that not only will they live longer than their parents but also that the infirmities afflicting so many elderly will never happen to them. In some cases they may be right, but life can be full of surprises, some of which can be prepared for and others that take every ounce of energy and resourcefulness to survive. The course our future will take will shift and change as we encounter new challenges, but we can plan for some of the possible pitfalls as a continuous exercise thus helping to manage fear of the unknown.

The problem comes when we cannot envision a time we will no longer be concentrating on the raising of our families, the pursuit of careers, or the effort to pull it all together to reach our dreams of success. In short, it is hard to think of retirement and beyond when one is used to focusing on the here and now but the fact is that strategic planning makes as much sense for us as it does for any successful business.

- Plan for the difficult times when we are active and vigorous.
- Learn how to communicate our hopes and expectations for the future to those closest to us.
- See that personal financial information and resources for spouses or relatives are available when they are needed.
- Challenge the theory that growing older has to mean growing lifeless.

Gee, You Don't Look 50, 60 or 70!

It's nice to hear someone say that, but I fail to understand what it means. What does 50, 60 or 70 look like? If we can get over the hurdle of decade counting and relating it to how old our parents seemed at the same age, we can begin to understand that we need not be limited by labels to get the most from what we choose to do. Aging is a matter of function rather than chronological steps in a preset plan. I haven't any idea how old I should look because each one of us ages in a unique way. I prefer to think that I am the way someone my age *should feel*. If I can stop thinking about aging as a time of unwelcome limits, then I can ignore how others think I should look and act at a certain age.

> *I haven't given much thought to how others see me or consider my age until one time looking through a house for sale with a realtor a few years ago. There were a lot of medicines lined up in the kitchen and items in the living room that led me to remark that the owners must be very old. The realtor replied that indeed they were as the husband was 64 years old. As I had just had my 64th birthday and didn't think of myself as old, I informed her I was the same age and "old" just wasn't the image I had of myself. Without pausing she assured me that she wasn't talking about a vibrant 64, she was referring to an old 64. Not a bad comeback and illustrates my point.*

Living Well is an Art Form

It seems to me that there is no artificial line to cross after which we must consider ourselves to be growing old; growing *older* perhaps, because by being alive we do that every day, every minute, every second. I feel we need never accept limitations without seeking other ways to reach out and embrace the good things life has to offer.

I have interviewed people in their 80s and 90s who have successfully maintained the ability to be independent. Common threads in each of their stories help explain why they seem so comfortable with their choices. One is a fierce determination to remain in control of their own lives, and another is a willingness to accept alternatives that may not have been consistent with what they would have preferred to do but which accommodated the possibility of future needs. They stayed involved in activities with other people and continued to travel to interesting places. Some exercised but others didn't. They all watched their diets with an eye to avoiding chronic or disabling conditions although none of them was fanatic about it. Three of the five people had moved from homes of many years into smaller apartments or "continuing care" communities where care is guaranteed according to the level of need for a lifetime. Two had considered it but they felt their present arrangements were adequate for their future needs.

All of them hoped that existing financial resources would be enough to maintain them no matter what their needs would be in the future, but none reassessed them on a regular basis. It occurred to each of them that changes in the provision of health care services and unexpected catastrophic medical emergencies could leave them penniless, but only one had had insurance policies evaluated by an objective expert to see if coverage had kept pace with rising costs.

What They Each Had in Common

Optimism: These people saw life as a feast from which they could pick and choose as they wished.

Flexibility: They never said never. Throughout their lives they accepted the fact that circumstances could require taking a different course than they had planned but saw no shame in changing their minds when it was called for.

Personal responsibility; They didn't waste a lot of time blaming someone else for things that went wrong.

Resilience; Traumatic and sad things had happened in most of their lives. The ability to work a way through them and even to find strength in surviving each one continued to give them confidence for the future.

A sense of purpose; When I asked one woman what her secret was, she said she always had a reason for getting up in the morning. Sometimes it took a little more effort to think what that reason was but when she went to bed at night she came up with something that made her look forward to the next day.

A healthy self-esteem; They value their own lives enough to care that they stay healthy and that they keep up with friends and relations. Personal appearance and home are maintained as a reflection of this sense of self.

So Where Does One Start?

There are many who share these qualities to some degree and who live into their 80s and 90s by balancing an understanding of their abilities and physical limitations with a desire to do more than move passively from one day to the next. Finding relevance in their stories may be difficult while we are in our middle years, but it is just that spirit which can lead us to start training ourselves now to make adjustments in the way we live our lives as we go along.

Strategies They Suggested

- Become knowledgeable about what we need to do to stay healthy.
- Set realistic goals for the maintenance of our health and personal welfare and make choices consistent with those goals.
- Reevaluate our positions physically, emotionally and financially at five-year intervals or after any life-changing event.
- Fight for the right to be flexible.
- Look for the formula that helps us to test and expand our minds.
- Enlarge our circle of friends to include all ages, younger and older.
- Cultivate and share a zest for living.
- Laugh at mistakes and learn from them.
- Whatever we do, we should do it with passion. The old cliche, "use it or lose it" is just as true with the mind as muscles.

Resource

I have found this book interesting, eye opening, and insightful about what is for some people a difficult subject to confront.

The Fountain of Age
By Betty Friedan—Simon & Schuster—1993—ISBN 0-671-40027-4

You Have to Know and Like Yourself to Move Successfully Into and Through any New Phase of Your Life.

Creating "arenas of respect" is another way of saying that we must learn how to like the person we have become. Using the strengths we have and exploring new ones helps us continue to move positively through life bringing co-workers, friends and relations along with us. Welcoming new skills or going back and exercising old ones keeps our minds active and healthy. Combining wisdom and experience with openness to new approaches for old problems keeps us flexible. In the future, when we perceive that physical changes, which limit our ability to enjoy our usual lifestyle have occurred, we are better able to find the energy and resolve to go around the obstacles and thus create a new life for ourselves.

Those who are generally regarded as successful, who are caring, productive and contributing members of their community are intimately aware of their capabilities and limits but are never hesitant to test them. They find respect without defining and demanding it. They are self-reliant but have also found value in the contributions of others to what they do.

People who are saddened by the end of a career, the sudden drawing in of horizons as the result of a traumatic injury or illness, or the loss of energy and sense of purpose that depression brings can lose sight of what has made them successful people. Success can be the achieving of small victories, the ability to draw strength from people met along the way and wisdom to learn from experience. Success is the ability to translate those elements into solutions to problems encountered and the completion of goals set for oneself.

The Secret To Problem Solving is Finding the Information and Services We Need

As our political and economic systems react to the aging "Baby Boomer" generation, voter and market pressures will force the creation of an increasing number of agencies and commercial enterprises to respond to their needs. There are retirement communities, assisted living, and senior housing communities; but finding the one we can afford, has the services we are looking for or the right atmosphere can be time consuming. Some of us will choose to renovate our homes and others to share a house or move in with a child. The process of selecting a favorable option requires planning, persistence, realistic self-knowledge and, once again, a willingness to be flexible.

There are resources provided by the federal government, states, counties and towns to help get services to those who need them. The trick is to know how to find them and this book should help you do that. Asking the right questions can lead to answers, which may not have been obvious at first. Some of the best clues to those questions can be found by comparing notes with friends who have already done the research and made their choices. Local newspapers, television documentaries and public radio programs often carry valuable information on subjects having to do with health, finances and "do it yourself" projects, such as how to make a home safer if failing eyesight or mobility becomes a problem.

Persistence is a Virtue.

In using some of the services specifically set up for the aging, I found polite, caring people who referred me to other people who sent me back to the people who couldn't help me in the first place. In one case, I was sent a list of organizations supposedly offering what I was looking for. There were twelve names on that list of which three were out of business, two didn't have the services as advertised; and the rest had waiting lists of a year or more. But with each phone call, I learned a little more and eventually found what I wanted.

If someone has mentioned a service is available in one city or town, asking for it in another will be easier. Phone numbers change, programs lose their funding and regulations in place today may not be there next year. Electronic answering systems and voice mail can be frustrating and never seem to cover one's specific needs; but Email and the Internet are tools that could facilitate the search. When able to speak to a human being on the phone, I have usually found the person is anxious to help if I state clearly what I am looking for and am willing to put in some time trying to help him or her help me. Keep in mind that services vary in different parts of the country and that one becomes more skilled in reaching a goal with experience.

Resource

The National Council on the Aging has a Website that helps the elderly and caregivers find out if they qualify for state and federal assistance programs.

www.benefitscheckup.org

If you don't use the Internet, call the local Agency on Aging to find a center that offers such a service

---

Use this as a workbook. Write notes and telephone numbers in the margins. When calling agencies or associations for help, write down the name of the person talked to, the date and a short synopsis of what that person said. When unable to find what is wanted, ask what other numbers can be called for further information. One lead will sometimes lead to another and often in circles, but eventually, if persistent enough, a solution can be found. Whether looking for answers for myself, or when I have been a caregiver for someone else, the skills used were the same.

Resource

I have used this service and found it to be helpful but not always perfect. It is at least a place to start looking for what is wanted. It is especially helpful if seeking help for someone who lives in another city or state as the resources are found by zip code.

ELDERCARE LOCATOR—1 800 677-1116

Social Security has a Web site offering information on Medicare, nursing homes, HUD housing and VA benefits as well as links to other services offered to the senior citizen.

www.seniors.gov

Using what our taxes have paid for makes good sense. Our tax dollars help to fund local, state and federal administrations that are there to provide information and services. By consulting with them, we are helping ourselves and also giving the organization an opportunity to justify its existence. Information from these agencies is often free to all comers and one should take advantage of their availability. Using the Internet, particularly with government agencies is often less frustrating than using the phone.

I never let labels stop me from asking for help. No one has refused to give me information because I did not fall into an appropriate age slot. "Elderly" or "senior citizen" means different things to different people and organizations. Although I think they are referring to someone a lot older than I am, it doesn't mean their information isn't useful.

Thinking About the Finale

The last chapter deals with the end of this life, as we know it. Many of us find it difficult to think about such an event, but if we are removed by age and good health from the immediacy of our own deaths, we can address the practical issues.

If aging begins the day we are born, we know from experience that it takes a long time when we are teenagers and moves a lot faster when we reach our middle years and beyond. Dying, although part of this natural process, becomes more relevant as we see it from the perspective of our own parents. Nothing else makes us think about how the journey will unfold for us more than their deaths. Throughout our adult lives we have learned to set our own goals, reviewed financial needs, plotted a course and then tried to make it happen. College, career, marriage, and raising children have brought uncertainties and surprises; planning for the middle years, very old age and beyond are no different. For example, having an up-dated will is good sense, but writing one's own obituary and planning whether we want a funeral or memorial service is the clearest expression of personal choice that can be made. The process can be very creative and even kind of interesting when looked at as an intellectual exercise.

> *We were listening to some wonderful music recently with friends and one of them said that he wanted his funeral to be filled with music. He became so enthusiastic about planning the event that he began then and there to select the music to be sung and played.*

CHAPTER TWO

RETIREMENT PLANNING
STARTS SOONER THAN WE THINK

I remember years ago going to an orientation given for the spouses of newly promoted admirals and listening to the first speaker welcome them with surprising words. He said, "Enjoy every moment of this affirmation of success and start, *this day*, to plan for your retirement." I now realize how valuable that advice was. A promotion with lives stretching before them and the wonder of new responsibilities . . . it was almost impossible to think that there could be any planning needed beyond the immediate future. He was a wise man as he had seen too often the way sudden turns and reverses could change a set course, and he knew the unhappiness of people who had not planned on making a life for themselves outside of their present career.

Popular wisdom was that Baby Boomers were so focused on the "right now" of life that they saw retirement as a stepping-stone to another career with more time to travel or do things with the family. Relatively young people, who only a few years ago were making unheard of salaries, are now out of a job. Millionaires at the age of 30 could not imagine a time when the good life might end, but many have to start over. They are not alone in being unwilling to think through what retirement and the later years will mean to them in terms of how their lives could change physically and financially. Studies have shown that many couples seriously underestimate the resources they would need to keep up their current standard of living. Many of the generation preceding us, my mother's contemporaries, lived through the Depression, the First and Second World War, and then lived in relative prosperity. But they also moved into their middle years and beyond with little understanding of how changing economics could affect their dreams for a worry free old age, which could be longer than they had anticipated.

The Care and Feeding of the Retired Business, Military, Medical, Corporate, and/or Compulsive Workaholic Person

Those who retire from a position of leadership in any field go from being the focal point, the final decision maker, and the place where "the buck stops," to feeling relatively irrelevant, often find it difficult to redefine themselves and redirect their sense of purpose when they leave the workplace. Experts in the field say that designing an exit strategy long before it is needed and making adjustments to it as one goes along are key factors in moving successfully into retirement. This does not imply that settling back and watching obligations be replaced by pleasant options does not make good sense. Welcoming choices that free time brings is also part of the planning. What I am suggesting is that entering retirement without some project in mind is like going to the supermarket without a list. You know you are there for a reason but can't think what it is and you waste a lot of time wandering around improvising.

In talking to friends who have recently retired from senior executive positions, I found it isn't the perks they miss the most. It is working with people from all walks of life who bring different skills together to benefit a larger purpose. There is a compelling reason for getting up every day but after retirement it is harder to redefine that sense of purpose. People who have translated an active workplace into a meaningful retirement have intuitively understood that principle and spent considerable time and effort planning what their next project or goal was going to be after the last day of work. Many of them have moved into challenging work on school boards or for political candidates, some into part-time consulting and others to volunteer with nonprofit organizations and still others into another full time career.

It is hard to imagine a time when the pace of daily challenges, the pressure to perform and out-perform ourselves will not be there. Retirement requires just as much strategic planning as any business proposition to take advantage of the freedom to choose what we want to do with the rest of our lives and to see that we have the resources to make it happen. It can be as simple as making a vow to read all the collected works of Charles Dickens, fish every salmon run in the US or as creative as writing the next great American novel. Retirement income may allow such indulgences but many feel the need to continue working for a salary to make up for the anticipated drop in income and to be prepared for emergencies down the road. My husband and I do not have full time jobs but we find that our projects still take more hours than there are in the day and although some are worthier than others they keep us interested and involved with other people.

For the Partner, Contemplating Retirement May Not be So Simple

Adjusting to retirement can take as much planning for the person who has never had a career outside the home as it does for one who has spent the largest number of waking hours in another workplace.

I, like many women of my generation, did not pursue a career after our children were born, sometimes managing the household alone for prolonged periods of time when my husband, a naval officer, was deployed at sea. At the same time, there were many of us "stay at home" wives who assisted other Navy families in need of support. None of us received a salary for our work, but it was as strong a commitment as to any career outside the home.

We raised our families, sent our children off to college, career and/or marriage, then moved into other pursuits to fill our days and use our energies productively. That freedom of choice in how we wished to spend our time, set within the usual parameters of any relationship involving more than one person, can become a jealously guarded right, a reward so to speak for all the years when time was not our own.

Some people whose spouses are approaching retirement, are apprehensive about the possible loss of relationships with other friends if moving is part of the equation. I sympathize because in military life, moving every two or three years meant we had to build new relationships frequently. The process was never easy, but as a result of those efforts, we now have friends all over the world who remain close to this day. We spent a lot of time going over the options and merits of many plans for what we wished to do with our lives after retirement and when the decision was said and done, we each felt that it was the best one

Making Adjustments

When my husband was close to retiring from the Navy, I listened with interest to the stories of those who had reached that point before us. I knew we would both have to learn a new set of rules for everyday living and that it could be difficult. We had each led a busy and rewarding life, were involved with many organizations, survived frequent long separations and were sometimes preoccupied with our own priorities. Our times together were usually peaceful and treasured but always with the understanding that they were interludes.

Friends warned me that for the first time in 34 years of marriage, I would lose the privilege of sorting through the mail every day. It doesn't sound like a big deal, but I was surprised how hard it is to have someone else decide what is junk mail and what isn't when I had been doing it for years. Still others spoke of the problem of making their own daily pastimes fit with proposals for living out retirement fantasies dreamed up by the retiree as the date neared. I found that problems with the use of the telephone became our biggest obstacle to marital peace. After several weeks of standing in line to make my phone calls and being distracted by an impatient husband consulting his watch while I talked to friends, we contracted for a second line. Every now and then, I have been reminded to put the complaints in perspective. When recounting my adventures to a friend, a recent widow, she wistfully said, "You're so lucky you have a husband to share retirement with."

I Married for Love. If It Means Lunch Too, So be It

We have all heard the saying this refers to and chuckled ruefully, but it reflects very real unease and nervousness about the way lives change for some married couples after retirement. If the marriage has followed the usual pattern of two people pursuing active careers and raising a family, the moments found to concentrate on each other may have been limited to vacation getaways or evenings out. From interviews with those recently retired and my own experience, I learned that togetherness takes a lot of getting used to. Even though there are plenty of projects to keep us busy, the natural result of spending so much time separated from each other will be the need to get to know one another all over again. Removing children from the equation because they have grown up and moved on finds us with increased leisure time and can reorder family dynamics more than we might expect.

Private space, both physical and emotional has been a lifesaver for us. Setting up a new division of labor in the running of our household took a lot more work and has ended up being more a negotiated settlement subject to frequent review, but it is working.

An engineer, John left his job at the mandatory retirement point in a very successful and long career. His wife, a lawyer, continued working full time in her own practice. Household chores that had largely been shared by the two of them now required a shift, as he was the one who had the time to assume responsibility for what is considered the unglamorous part of running a household. In his acceptance of the requirement to keep the house stocked with food and necessaries, he went about it with an engineer's mind. Coupons were clipped and filed and the marketing list was a direct reflection of those items. His wife relates that the freezer is full of more ice cream novelties than she knew existed and the pantry is stocked with bottles and boxes of every cleaning substance and plastic bag advertised. When the freezer gets too full to cram anything else in, and the pantry reaches the saturation point, she quietly carries the excess to her children who live in their own households nearby. The local supermarket cashiers awarded him a prize for the neatest and most organized cart in the store!

An amusing story, but it also illustrates two points. He has taken on a job many men who grew up in our generation would be reluctant to accept. He has welcomed going into what could be considered an alien environment by applying skills second nature to him. His wife may feel that he hasn't quite got it right yet, but wisely, she is not discouraging his zeal or his desire to contribute.

Retirement as a Springboard to Opportunity

Retirement, if it occurs in middle age, coincides for some women who are not working outside the home, with a rush of energy and sense of purpose. After the responsibilities of raising a family shift, and children take their active lives somewhere else, they readjust to independence; they begin to envision doing something for themselves. Many reenter the workplace as corporate lawyers, psychiatrists, social workers, political appointees, financial managers, and published authors. Others go back to creative pursuits long delayed by careers and other things. Sometimes called *post-menopausal adolescence*, it describes my feelings at this time in my life as being full of enthusiasm and energy, as I break out of the usual molds by testing limits previously encountered by my husband's career requirements and raising a family.

Resource

I found this compelling reading years ago and still go back to it to find how well she puts into words what I understood only vaguely before. I have read conflicting reviews of the book but still think that it has valuable insights.

New Passages, Mapping your Life Across Time
By Gail Sheehy—Random House—1995—ISBN 0-394-58913-0

"Come Age with Me. The Best is Yet to be." Robert Browning

There are many people facing retirement who want that to be true but aren't sure how to make it happen. An idyllic retirement as viewed by the person who wants to live it means something different to each one of us. We are all aware that successful relationships take work and frequent realignment. The trouble is that some of us are better at it than others. We have had experience in making adjustments through courtship, marriage, career moves, parenting, and, if children have been a presence up until now, becoming a twosome after they move away. Retirement calls for awakening those skills once again.

When a partner retires, some of us find that we become supporter and cheerleader for a person who is restructuring a life outside the needs of going to work every day. At the same time, we may feel that our own needs are not being considered. Those of us who have given any thought to retirement, realize that the equation for a balanced marriage changes and grows as circumstances dictate and that this is another one of those times when communication and forethought encourage better understanding. The ability to welcome this new stage comes from drawing on what it was that made us want to be together in the first place and what we have become as individuals and partners in the years since then.

LOVE is a Four Letter Word

With demands made on a marriage by careers, raising a family and the hectic pace of trying to keep up with the rush of such a life, moving from the usual and well-traveled paths in our lives is difficult. Some of us don't recognize that warmth and intimacy have taken a back seat until the children have gone or retirement has started and we are faced with the prospect of discovering who we have become in the intervening years. For those who have enjoyed a satisfying and healthy sex life full of commitment, the possibility that it could become even deeper and more meaningful as we age may not have occurred to us as we contemplated retirement.

I am no expert on sex for the aging person, but I have done research on the subject for this book and am heartened to discover what I had suspected to be the case is backed by those knowledgeable in the field. What is clear is that, if sex was important when we were younger then it will be when we are 70 or older. Although stages of sexual response may take longer than when we were younger, making love should be no less fulfilling and hopefully more so as we find the time and freedom to express it. What is also clear is that health and fitness are as important factors in an active and satisfying sex life as are the brain and "the heart". It is the relearning of signals for intimacy and the reconnection of that "hands on" approach that becomes the path for creating a new atmosphere. It is very hard to keep from comparing oneself to images of sensuality and sexuality we see in movies and television but the fact is that we have an opportunity to write a new chapter in our relationships and to keep adding others as we go on.

Some of us will come up against health problems that have an impact on our desire and ability to enjoy sex as we have always known it. We should know that medication prescribed for another condition could be causing problems and that there are solutions to such conditions as erectile dysfunction and decreased sexual desire. Women may find intercourse uncomfortable after menopause but a doctor can assist with solutions to that problem as well.

If we have not learned how to express our concerns to each other, now is the time to begin. When problems occur, people often give up touching, hugging and caressing for fear of being unable to follow through. That intimate contact is now more necessary than it ever was. The fact is that the whole body is a sensory organ and there are many other deeply satisfying ways to give and receive pleasure. Learning how together is the reward we get for caring about each other.

Know What Questions to Ask About Retirement

What if he wants to move to Minnesota and I hate cold weather?
What if he wants me home all the time with him and I have other things to do?
What if she wants to travel and I just want to enjoy being home?
What if we don't like each other when we have to spend a lot of time together?
What if she is tired of the "rat race" and I still enjoy it?
What if he wants me to give up my job?
What if we don't have enough income to retire?
What if illness strikes? Will we have enough to pay the bills?
What if I die? Will my partner have enough to live on?
What if I am single and my pension isn't enough to cover present expenses?

This is the Time for Refining the Skill of "Horse Trading"

Those questions present a set of challenges for each partner when giving in, giving up and giving back may be more difficult than imagined.

In reviewing options for our own retirement, I learned a great deal about this person I had been living with for so many years. When we were able to focus on the issue we found a lot more we agreed on than disagreed. Several years later the learning has not stopped.

We had been told that building a house together would be the ultimate test of our relationship. He was an engineer by training with the ability to visualize things from a blueprint, which I had expected. Since this is not a skill of mine, he had to come up with a way make me see what was so clear to him. He also wanted to be included in the creative design decisions that I had thought would be mine to make; and although I felt he was moving into my territory, I found he brought a lot of good ideas to the process. We had little trouble settling on a place to retire, but coming to agreement on the details required a great deal more negotiation. The "getting there" was not easy but it taught me a lot about us and we ended up with what we both wanted in the end.

- Find a time and location where serious conversations can be held without interruptions. I found the automobile to be the best venue because there were no phones, (no cell phones), no TV, and few distractions.
- Set priorities independently, and compare them. I was surprised how many we agreed on.
- We both thought about what we liked most about our lives and what we wanted to give up least.
- We tried to express those thoughts in a non-confrontational and non-judgmental way. (This is the hardest one)
- I learned to compromise on the small things and saved my energy for the big ones.
- If communication has not been a strong suit, find ways to improve it. One of the most difficult things for people to learn in any partnership is how to balance communication needs. I solve problems by talking about them to the point of exhaustion. My husband doesn't see as many problems as I do and doesn't need all the input to work out what he does see. We need to recognize that people process

information differently. We're working on it, but habits of a lifetime are hard to break.
- We took the time to review and reevaluate our financial resources to prepare for retirement. Becoming suddenly single will painfully illustrate how not talking about financial issues over the years can mean drowning in a sea of uncertainties and worries if a partner should die.

Resource

This is an easy to read, clear explanation of the need for women to become knowledgeable about financial matters that directly impact their lives. Men may find it equally as valuable.

Prince Charming Isn't Coming How Women Get Smart About Money
By Barbara Stanney—Penguin USA—1999—ISBN 0140266933

Being Single Makes Planning for Retirement Less Complicated but Not Easier

For those of us living alone, the questions remain the same. Planning one's future without having to consider the wishes of a partner may be less complicated, but it also is more difficult to find a focus when the job is over. It is for this reason that we need to give some thought to what we will do with our lives after retirement. Building a new life, strengthening friendships, and renewing ties with relatives are just a few of the pleasures of having more free time. These old/new relationships are an investment in a support system for the future but equally important, they give the opportunity to think beyond the confines of job and home. The most important emphasis is to be planning for a time when one might be incapacitated. Being alone narrows our options.

CHAPTER THREE

A Healthy Attitude May be the Best Medicine

If the proliferation of health and fitness magazines is any indication, more of us are making life-affirming decisions to improve lifestyle and longevity with exercise and better nutrition. In this way the responsibility for staying healthy is beginning to shift from a burden carried by the doctor alone to a more equitable sharing of the load by patient and doctor.

We are also changing the way we seek medical help. Pharmaceutical companies are marketing prescription drugs directly to the public, counting on individuals to pressure their doctors into prescribing them and it has been profitable. There is increasing concern that antibiotics, as we know them can no longer control many of the virulent, disease causing bacteria because of overuse. Increased advertising for "Natural" products, news reports of the multi-billion dollar nutritional supplement business and the proliferation of practitioners of alternative therapies gives a clear picture of the disillusionment many people have with the old way of practicing medicine.

Acupuncture, naturopathy, Chinese herbal medicine, homeopathy, bee sting therapy, chiropractic, therapeutic energy, and massage therapy have emerged from relative obscurity to acceptance by a public newly conscious of the sometimes serious side effects of powerful drugs on the complex systems of the body. The process of curing symptoms with dangerous drugs, while saving lives, often does irreparable damage to otherwise healthy organs.

Doctors trained in traditional medicine are using therapies from other cultures as another tool to ease human suffering rather than perceiving them to be a threat to the medicine they had been taught in medical school. There are an increasing number of doctors who use holistic medicine, treatment of the whole person rather than alleviating symptoms of a specific condition, and there are others who use a combination of traditional and complementary medicine. Dr. Andrew Weil is a well-known example of a doctor/practitioner who has brought the best of both types of medicine to a public increasingly looking for alternatives to what they have always known. Finding and evaluating them is not easy but as the demand grows, so will the availability. The clearest sign of growing acceptance is that this type of treatment is often called *complementary* or *integrative* medicine rather than *alternative*.

Although many health insurance plans at this writing do not cover such approaches, they will in time as they are proving to be more cost effective. Regrettably, there are presently no standards by which herbal medicines and other "natural" substances are measured in the USA, as some of them can be hazardous to one's health. The American Medical Association is calling for scientific evaluation of these therapies so the public can be more certain of their efficacy. There is now a National Center for Complementary and Alternative Medicine, which is currently funding studies on many aspects of alternative treatments. Until a system for evaluating practitioners and therapies comes along, we will have to rely on word of mouth, reputation and good common sense to find the best source.

A Nutritionist Should be Your New Best Friend

As we learn how important nutrition is in maintaining good health, it becomes clear that some doctors are unfamiliar with the importance of all aspects of nutrition as a health tool. In many cases doctors do not receive thorough training in medical school about the effects of vitamin and mineral deficiency on many illnesses and the complexity of interaction of drugs, nutritional supplements and herbal remedies.

A **nutritionist**, on the other hand, is a specialist who has been trained in how the body functions, how nutrients are absorbed and metabolized and how they interact with other nutrients as well as drugs. This requires a thorough knowledge of graduate level biochemistry, physiology and other scientific course work. Nutritionists must have an advanced degree from an accredited college or university and should be certified by the Certification Board for Nutrition Specialists of the American College of Nutrition. The CNS (Certified Nutrition Specialist) designation following the name means that person has received proper training and a masters or doctoral degree in nutrition sciences. With the proliferation of food supplements and new medicines, theories on what to eat to stay healthy and what to avoid are difficult to follow. Advice from such a professional is invaluable in any strategy for good health.

Resource

A service of Tufts University, this is a Website providing a guide to nutrition sites and rates them for accuracy and usefulness. Up-dated quarterly, it is easy to read and informative. It is a service of Tufts University.

www.navigator.tufts.edu

This USDA Food and Nutrition Information Center has many resources and information on all aspects of nutrition including vitamins and supplements.

www.nal.usda.gov/fnic

A dietician is trained in designing a regimen of special or limited food and drink for those whose condition requires it. Usually operating in food service but also in clinical areas, especially in institutions such as schools, nursing homes or hospitals, this professional has training in tailoring standard diets to medical or dietary restrictions. The certifying Board affiliated with the American Dietetic Association offers the designation RD (Registered Dietician), indicating completion of training at the undergraduate level.

A Geriatric Specialist Can Save Your Life

Most doctors who specialize in geriatrics have a clear understanding of the unique differences in the aging metabolism and take a holistic and preventive approach to treating health problems. Their task is to find the best way to manage illness while helping the patient to function at the best level possible. In other words, they manage chronic conditions where no cure is possible. Their training and experience makes them aware of the difficulty in maintaining proper levels of medication in the elderly who may have concurrent medical problems for which they are receiving different drugs. That knowledge could, for example, reverse symptoms of pseudodementia and even save lives.

Not everyone over the age of 65 needs a gerontologist, nor should the name of the specialty keep one from taking advantage of the service before they are 65. We all want doctors who will evaluate us as individuals and who recognize our unique characteristics and requirements.

> *After abdominal surgery for cancer, my mother had a common, non-life-threatening but uncomfortable urinary tract infection. A call to her primary physician, an internist she had consulted for many years, referred us to her surgeon who prescribed medication in a dosage that would have been appropriate for a younger adult of average age and weight. She was 84 years old and weighed 90 pounds. When she had seizures, both doctors attributed it to the spread of her original disease. It was only at the suggestion of a doctor friend who guessed her kidneys were*

not clearing the medicine from her body that we understood she was being systematically overdosed to toxic levels. Her doctor had not taken into consideration her age or weight. We suspended her medication and her seizures stopped.

Resource

To help in your search for a doctor trained in geriatric medicine in your area, call the number below and they will send you a list of specialists in your state.
 The American Geriatrics Society—Toll free—1 866 788-3939

Getting in the Mood

Kenneth Pelletier, in his book, *Sound Mind, Sound Body,* says that the pursuit of good health should be "an ongoing process of self-discovery". Understanding the changes that are occurring naturally to our bodies, finding ways to prevent the troubling ones, and pushing ourselves to stay involved with other people in a way, which stimulates the mind, are only the beginning. He tells us that in order to put in place a lifelong plan for good health, we must combine physical, mental, spiritual and quality of life strategies and then have the discipline to embrace them as a way of life. There have been countless documented stories of spontaneous remissions of desperate illness that cannot be explained scientifically. Concurrently, doctors are beginning to understand that a patient's driving will to live may be the most valuable tool there is in the battle to get well and stay well.

Resource

The author makes his point in a clear, easy to read manner by interviewing well-known role models.
 Sound Mind, Sound Body: A New Model for Lifelong Health
 By Dr. Kenneth R. Pelletier—Simon and Schuster—ISBN: 067 177 0004

Why Bother?

Barring chronic or catastrophic illness, accident or addiction to health destroying substances, living longer and healthier means we must learn to take better care of our bodies. Statistics tell me that if I reach the age of 70 in relatively good health, my total *active life expectancy* will continue to grow, thus I have a good chance of moving into the next decade and beyond with an acceptable quality of life.

What the numbers don't tell us is that choosing to lead a healthy life-style involves a lot of work. Learning how to make a new system of health care deliver the services we feel we deserve and being a better-informed medical consumer are skills that we will have to learn. We will need to learn how to listen to and understand the signals our body sends us and take a common sense approach to weight control, exercise and eating habits. Evaluating the doctor and getting a second and third opinion when surgery or treatment requiring potent drugs is recommended is an important part of the equation. Learning about integrative (alternative) medicine or therapy and how to find the best practitioners requires research skills. Knowledge brings confidence; fueling the energy and the will we must have for doing what it takes to stay healthy.

Maybe We Should Call It the Fountain of Life!

Ken Dychtwald, in an article on longevity in the *Washington Post Magazine* referred to those who are experiencing long, productive lives as people who are "growing old agelessly". The increasing number of people some think of as "really old", (in their 80's or 90's), who continue to work full or part-time and who seek out opportunities for new and creative pursuits don't think of retirement as a time to step back from their active lives. They have defined a purpose in life that consumes their interest, and have followed through with focused energy. This positive, activist attitude is what it takes to help view aging as a time to discover its treasures.

Recently I heard a friend my age say to someone younger, "Don't grow old, it's just a series of aches and pains." She truly believes that and the more she says it the more it becomes fact for her. Worse, it raises expectations that everyone has to feel the same way when they reach a certain age. I understand there are times in life when it could take too much energy to make the effort and that the frailties of an uncooperative body make one wonder if it is worth pressing on. What I have discovered from my interviews is that surviving the down times and pushing ourselves to find solutions to blows, which sometimes seem to come in endless procession, gives us strength to carry on. The loss of long time friends our own age can sometimes leave us feeling lonely and increasingly isolated especially if living alone. Drawing on the store of strength built up through experience and wisdom by encouraging friendships of all ages has helped one 90-year-old friend through those bad moments. There may be a time in the future of slowing down and accepting limitations for this person but she has taught me that if we exploit those skills gained over the years and reflect on how to enjoy them it will be because we have trained ourselves to do so.

Resource

This is one of the most complete and interesting resource books for women, I have found. I go back to it again and again because of its positive approach. There is a 1997 edition but harder to find than the one listed below.
THE NEW OURSELVES, GROWING OLDER A Book for Women Over Forty
Women Aging with Knowledge and Power
By Paula B. Doress-Worters and Diana Laskin Siegal

In cooperation with The Boston Women's Health Book Collective—Simon & Schuster—1994—ISBN 0-671-87297-4

Staying Healthy
By Learning About The Changing Body

One way to stay healthy is to learn how to interpret the signals our body sends us. I recognize that changes have been occurring to my body during my lifetime but I have become more sensitive to them as I perceive them to be signs of growing old. My hair doesn't seem as thick and full as it once was and I don't need a deodorant as often. Where once I could sleep through the night without a problem, now getting up once or twice to use the bathroom is standard practice. I used to be able to eat anything and everything without a second thought, but now find myself avoiding dairy foods and extra spicy items.

With the help of a friend knowledgeable about these things, I have been trained in self-awareness and have a better understanding of what is happening. I have a better idea when to seek help for a more serious condition and how to restore the natural balance of my body when there are problems. Learning what to expect, and accepting that some of what is happening is because the body's needs are changing makes us more sensitive to the adjustments that have to be made to our former way of life. I have friends who want to know whether all the effort to stay fit and healthy is worth it when conventional wisdom tells us that we add only days or a week to our longevity. I am convinced that by finding the right formula for good health I am prolonging the time I feel wonderful, not just extending my life.

When I was 10 or 11 years old and growing inches in days, I remember complaining about pains in my legs as bones and muscles struggled to keep up with the growth imperative. Now many of us wake up in the morning complaining of pain in lots of those same places. It's not from growing taller; it's apt to be from strains placed on the body for other reasons, like being overweight, lack of exercise or the beginning of chronic health problems brought about by stress. I can't guarantee that leading a healthier lifestyle will make all those pains magically disappear. If we educate ourselves, and have the follow-through to put what we learn into action, we will move through life feeling as though *we* are making the choices, rather than an ailing and weakening body doing it for us. Some illnesses or infirmities require more energy and courage to overcome than others. Even the most severe problems can be endured if we assert a wish to be in control of our own health decisions and thereby live our lives proactively rather than passively accepting everything that comes our way.

Resource

This is a much-needed reference for men from AARP. I am getting one for my husband and keeping it as a reference for both of us. I have found all their guides well presented and covering a lot of the issues.
 Staying Strong: For Men Over Fifty: A Common Sense Guide (D15296)
  Address a postcard to:—AARP Fulfillment, (EE0858)—
   601 E St. NW
   Washington, DC 20049

I have reviewed a number of newsletters and have found this a most complete and balanced presentation. It is a great way to keep up with advances in good health and to get an overview of health issues expressed from many points of view.
Subscription Information—UC Berkeley Wellness Newsletter—Tel: 1 904 445-6414
   PO Box 420148
   Palm Coast, FLA 32142

Some Examples of What our Bodies are Trying to Tell Us

 The first thing to remember is that each of us will age at our own rate and in our own way. Everyone's body chemistry is unique, and therefore, any discussion of body changes will have to take that individuality into account. There are some common denominators. Experts feel that many troubling aspects of the aging process are caused by nutritional deficiencies, lack of regular exercise and changes in hormonal balance, which many of us have the ability to reverse. Their premise is that research has shown us that life care decisions, like giving up smoking, keeping weight under control and having regular medical check-ups are indications that we are unwilling to accept limitations as part of the aging process we have been led to believe is inevitable.

Hair: Diminishing blood supply to the scalp causes hair to grow more slowly, perhaps to become thinner and change texture. Baldness, particularly in the male, may be inherited, but in both male and female could be from other causes that, with treatment, might be reversed. Hair may start to gray because the body is producing less color pigment.

Course of action: Hair loss may occur with thyroid malfunction or if one's diet is vitamin or mineral deficient. Increase circulation to the scalp with massage but beware of "snake oil" treatments. (Big promises, little action) Ask a hairdresser or barber if the shampoo being used could be causing the problem and whether a new haircut by a skilled person can mask or alleviate it. Graying of the hair is probably on a genetic timetable so the best course may be to grin and bear it.

Kidney and bladder: Kidney function and filtration rate drop as blood flow in the kidneys slows. Less efficient function occurs naturally as one ages causing toxins and medicines to remain in the body longer. Kidneys are key to the elimination of wastes and poisons, (including medication), therefore the effect of drugs on the body may be exaggerated as a person ages. Bladder capacity declines requiring more frequent elimination and loss of pelvic muscle tone can result in urinary incontinence. Discolored urine may indicate infection but could also be the result of something eaten, like beets, or could be caused by the ingestion of some vitamins, minerals or medications. Blood in the urine, even if transitory demands the attention of a physician.

Course of action: When taking a prescription for other conditions, the doctor and/or pharmacist should be aware of our age and weight, both of which can affect the speed with which substances are cleared from the system. Whether currently having problems with incontinence or not, ask the doctor about Kegel exercises and do them regularly. Drink more water during the day but no later than three hours before bedtime and consider the possibility that a medication taken for another condition, including some vitamin supplements can affect urination. Men should see their doctors if they have difficulty in urinating, frequency or burning to check for possible prostate or bladder disease.

Bones: Osteoporosis primarily affects post-menopausal women, but also affects men, particularly those who are thin and slightly built. The condition becomes apparent later in men than women because they usually have denser bones to start with. Gradual demineralization causes loss of bone mass, therefore increasing chance of bone fractures, loss of height and "dowager's hump" due to fractures of the vertebrae. There is also a condition called osteomalacia, which is a disease affecting bone caused by lack of Vitamin D. Levels of Vitamin D in the body can be increased by being exposed to the sun for 15 minutes each day from April to October. With the fear of skin cancer keeping a lot of people out of the sun or covered in sunscreen, this is becoming an increasingly common problem.

Course of action: Menopausal women should consult a doctor for an appropriate preventative program particularly if they fall into the high-risk group for osteoporosis. A balanced diet sometimes requiring supplements such as calcium and other important minerals and vitamins is recommended together with a regular exercise regimen of weight bearing and resistance exercises developed by a trained therapist. Exposure to some sun each day helps the body absorb Vitamin D which in turn helps one to assimilate and retain calcium.

Vision: Night vision becomes less acute, color perception decreases and the possibility of cataracts increases after the age of 65. Vision problems for those who have not had them before can begin in the 40s and a decrease in ability to see fine details can occur in the 70s with macular degeneration being one of the most serious. Some drugs can cause vision impairment; therefore any changes should be reported to the doctor when taking a new medication.

Course of action: Regular examinations by an eye doctor for signs of glaucoma and other serious eye diseases, and consultation with a nutritionist for supplements are recommended. Check also with the eye doctor for the best type of sunglasses to avoid exposure to the harmful effects of bright sunshine, ultraviolet rays and low-level radiation such as x-rays.

Hearing: High frequency hearing loss and resulting tinnitus, (persistent ringing or buzzing in the ear) are not infrequent problems facing people who have had excessive exposure to loud noise for a prolonged period of time. High blood pressure can also cause ringing in the ears.

Course of action: Wearing ear protectors when operating loud machinery and lowering the volume of sound equipment will minimize future damage. A specialist should check hearing. Have blood pressure checked regularly.

Taste and smell: Taste and smell decline gradually after the age of 40 and by 50% after 65 or could come from the effect of certain medications.

Course of action: Giving up smoking is one way to improve the problem. Consult a nutritionist to see if it could be the result of a vitamin deficiency.

RESOURCE

I tried this screening number and it worked for me. It is obviously not as good as a trip to the doctor but it does give one a good indication that a more thorough evaluation by a professional may be needed.

Dial a Hearing Screening Test—Monday through Friday 9 AM-5 PM Eastern Time—800 222 3277

Teeth and gums: Pain during chewing, bleeding gums, loose teeth and halitosis are all signs of gingivitis and periodontal disease.

Course of action: Regular removal of plaque by a dentist is recommended along with a regimen of daily dental flossing, brushing and strict attention to diet with emphasis on foods, which stimulate the gums. Vitamin and mineral supplements are sometimes suggested in addition to the dental attention. My advisor explained that gum disease can be a sign of scurvy, the ancient sailor's curse, thus some people have had success taking increased doses of Vitamin C and other supplements. Changing the toothbrush at least once a month and using a dentifrice or toothpaste containing ingredients to help prevent bacterial action on the gums will also help. Heavy smoking and alcohol consumption can also cause problems. If having surgery be sure to notify the surgeon, if you have gum disease or gingivitis because it could affect recovery.

Resource

This Web site has very good information on women's health issues including oral health and how it relates to overall health. They will send a free copy of: "The Women's Guide to Oral Health". Tel: 1 877 986—9472

www.healthywomen.org

High blood pressure: Arteries may be obstructed by a buildup of plaque causing the heart to work harder to push blood through a narrower opening and thereby elevating blood pressure.

Course of action: A doctor or nutritionist can give guidelines for a healthy, well balanced diet to go along with prescribed medicine. Eat fresh foods rather than processed and "fast" foods. Low sodium intake may help, but some salt is necessary for normal body function. Many doctors will suggest regular exercise if weight is a problem as it can be dangerous to anyone with high blood pressure.

Skin: The appearance of wrinkles, spots and/or bumps is a clue that skin is aging. As a natural by-product of this process, fat is redistributed from under the skin to deeper parts of the body. Skin loses its elasticity, is thinner and becomes increasingly dry causing it to flake and appear more fragile.

Course of action: Regular exercise prevents loss of lean body tissue and helps maintain skin tone. Drinking plenty of water and avoiding direct exposure to the sun without proper sunscreen products helps slow down wrinkling and dryness of the skin. Smoking has been shown to cut down on oxygen delivery to cells in the skin and soft drinks and junk food are thought to cause problems as well.

Resource

I have used this book often for minor problems and found that it is practical and helpful. It is up-dated and republished now and then.

Prescription for NUTRITIONAL HEALING, A Practical A-Z Reference To Drug-Free Remedies Using Vitamins, Minerals, Herbs and Food Supplements.
By James F. Bach, M.D. and Phyllis A. Bach, C.N.C.
Avery—Penguin Putnam Inc.—2000—ISBN 1-58333-077-1

So Many New Theories, Therapies and Puzzles to Sift Through

As mentioned earlier, researchers and doctors who study the effects of aging are attempting to reduce the onset of chronic disability and decline through the use of lifestyle changes and medical advances. Some are attempting to alter the way our bodies mature by halting or reversing degeneration of the body's cells. Surgery to remove cataracts has brought clear sight to millions of people and the replacement of damaged joints has relieved pain and increased mobility for many arthritis sufferers.

Gene engineering and therapy hold much promise for the future. Hormone replacement therapy (HRT) for women although prescribed for many years to relieve some effects of menopause and slowing of the loss of bone mass, showed early promise of lowering the risk of heart attack and in some cases preventing or delaying the effects of Alzheimer's in some people. Recently there have been some serious questions raised and studies reported that suggest those benefits may be exaggerated and may not outweigh the increased risk of heart attack, breast cancer and stroke. Stay tuned. Vitamin and mineral supplements are increasingly being embraced as a way to stay healthy physically and emotionally.

How we receive health information has changed from conferences with the doctor to the addition of what we can glean from the mass media and find for ourselves on the Internet. Trying to keep up with all the information is difficult enough. Knowing what is fraudulent while recognizing what is valuable is becoming increasingly difficult requiring more diligent investigation by the consumer.

Eating Well Can Help Keep us Well

One of the things I have learned, in an attempt to pick my way through the different things I read about nutrition, is that what is healthy for me may not be the best thing for someone else. There are several points to keep in mind when consulting those RDA guidelines. When the government lists requirements of certain nutrients for a proper diet, it is based on an average person rather than adjusting for individual needs. It does not take into consideration the fact that each body may have different dietary requirements; therefore following it strictly may cause one person to gain weight and another to lose it.

Resource

Prevention Magazine listed a number of what they felt were the best Web sites for reliable, useful information on nutrition. For one of the most comprehensive and downright fun sites try this.—*www.mealsforyou.com*

If you are confused by information in newspapers, magazines and on television about what the USDA recommends as a daily diet to maintain good health for most people, (excepting sedentary adults, active teenagers, etc.), you are like most of us. Requirements change frequently and by the time this book is printed would probably have changed once again so we follow the advice of the doctor or nutritionist for what will work best for our body, then keep reading and evaluating the latest theories and make decisions as we go along. So many factors influence what diet is the best for each individual that following one set of guidelines could never cover everyone. Chronic disease, genetic make-up, food allergies, your family background and ethnic, religious or moral beliefs and personal tastes are only some. If you are trying to lose weight like so many of us, find the diet plan that works best for you and remember that the key ingredient in any successful plan is increasing the amount of exercise you do on a daily basis.

Many of us Eat Too Much

Obesity is becoming a major health problem in the US. Part of the problem is that we eat too much and exercise too little. For the sake of clarification, I include what the government refers to as a serving size so that when consulting a diet plan, you can have a better idea of how much food they are talking about. The best advice then is to be guided by the proportion of grains to protein, etc. as indicated and to count calories if trying to lose weight. People who are limited in the exercise they can do should be cutting down on the amount of food they eat.

For an Idea of What is called a Serving Size

Pasta/bread—1 serving = 1\2 cup cooked or 4 twirls of the fork, I slice of bread

Meat—1 serving = 2-3 ounces (A serving of meat in a restaurant may be 3—4 times larger than that

Fruit—1 serving = ¾ cup juice, (6 oz.)

Vegetable—1 serving = 1 c. raw vegetables such as salad, ½ c. cooked

RESOURCE

My favorite Web site on nutritional matters, I have found that they have 8 "pyramids" indicating different types of healthful diets with foods one should eat least of at the top and unlimited types on the bottom.

www.mayoclinic.com

Give Red Meat a Chance

Lowering the amount of animal, (saturated) fat we eat is currently accepted as a way to prevent several diseases. "Marbling," the lacing of lean meat with fat, has become a bad word. Although eating red meat without guilt is a thing of the past until another study tells us differently, nutritionists say there are reasons why we should not give it up entirely.

Research from Utah State University indicates that people who avoid eating red meat may not be getting enough iron and many people view fish, and white meat chicken as leaner and healthier. Keep in mind that chicken, meat and some farm raised fish are fed hormones and antibiotics, which when we consume them is added to our diets and thus may be harmful to us. The consumption of red meat has declined 14% since 1975. The popularity of poultry has tripled and fish has increased about 20% since 1960 leading to the conclusion that consumers may be overlooking the importance of meat as a good source of iron.

70% of all foods are processed before being sold. This degrades an easily absorbable type of iron into a form the body does not take in as well. For instance, chicken breast has only 8% and chicken legs only 32% of the type of iron found in the same amount of cooked ground beef. Keep in mind that red meat is a protein that can supply not only iron, but also zinc and vitamins B/6 and B/12. If one chooses lean cuts such as eye of the round, top round and top sirloin, 6 oz. of red meat holds no more saturated fat than the same amount of chicken.

Reading the Labels—"Lite" is Not Necessarily Low Fat or Low Calorie

With all the emphasis on "eating healthy" these days, finding one's way through labeling for nutritional guidelines can be daunting. "Lite" or "Light" does not necessarily mean that a product is lower in calories. It means that by Federal law it must contain at least 1/3 fewer calories or 1/2 the fat of the original product. *Read the label carefully.* Sugar free or sugarless means what it says; no sugar, no corn syrup and no fructose. Low or reduced calories means that the product has 1/3 fewer calories than something of the same type. This may not mean less fat nor does it mean that the calorie count is what would qualify it as a diet food. *Read the label carefully.*

Common Sense and a Little Knowledge Help the Labels Help Us

Nutrition labels are not difficult to understand once they have been explained. I don't always read them completely but I do consult them regularly. I look for the serving size, the calories, the ingredients, the total fat and its breakdown into different types of fat, the sodium content, sugars and fiber.

Ingredients are Listed in Descending Order of Percentage of the Total

For example, the ingredients in ginger cookies are listed on the box as follows;

- Enriched wheat flour, [wheat flour, niacin, reduced iron, thiamine mononitrate (vitamin B1), riboflavin, (vitamin B2), folic acid]. It is the first ingredient listed therefore has the greatest volume, and although it lists vitamins and minerals, they are not added unless so noted but are natural characteristics of wheat flour.

- Sugar, molasses, vegetable shortening (partially hydrogenated soybean and/or canola oils)
- High fructose corn syrup, ginger, baking soda, salt, and oil of lemon.
- Sugar, molasses and high fructose corn syrup are sweeteners.
- The percentages listed as %Daily Value, mean that the ingredients listed are a percentage of a 2000-calorie diet. They fulfill a percentage of what the US Department of Agriculture feels are the minimum daily needs of the average body for healthy function.

If cutting down on the amount of sugar consumed, or worried about how fattening a product is, check to see what constitutes a serving size, (the amount from which the nutritional figures are drawn) and then the number of calories in that amount. The serving size in this case is 7 cookies that would add 130 calories to the diet.

The Nutrition Facts label required on processed foods, gives a breakdown of what those ingredients mean nutritionally. I have already mentioned the serving size and calories. Now the label will tell what percentage of calories are from fat and what types of fat they are.

> Total Fat 4.5g = 7%
> Saturated fat—1 g, (gram) = 5%
> Polyunsaturated fat = 0g
> Monounsaturated fat = 2g

Now we get to the hard part. Words that are guaranteed to make my eyes glaze over are the ones listed under total fats. My rule of thumb used to be that if there are more than two ingredients I don't recognize or can't pronounce then I don't want to consume the product, but it really is more complicated than that. Here is a short explanation.

Saturated fat is the visible fat on beef, pork and the dark meat of chicken. Butter, egg yolk, some dairy foods, palm and coconut oils are other sources.

Monounsaturated fats are olive, peanut, rice bran and canola oils.

Polyunsaturated fats are from vegetables such as sunflowers, safflower, soybean and corn as well as fish like salmon, tuna and mackerel.

Hydrogenated fats, (not listed on this label) are solidified, unsaturated fats such as those found in margarine, packaged crackers, cookies and other store bought baked goods. These contain many *Trans-fatty acids* that may have started as unsaturated liquid oils but have been processed to change their chemical structure. These Trans-fats raise levels of the waxy cholesterol that clog our blood vessels and lower the amount of the "good" cholesterol we have. There is emerging evidence that they can raise the infection processes, which may lead to heart disease and cancer. Stick margarine contains fatty acids, which allows it to hold its shape whereas the tub margarine has water that is substituted for the fat.

Not All Fats are Bad

Fats contain essential nutrients and allow cells in the body to function properly. The problem comes from consuming too much fat particularly if it is the wrong type. Just because a product is low in fat, does not necessarily mean that it is better. It does not do any good to load up on low fat cookies because the listing indicates only a few grams of fat. If it is a highly processed product containing hydrogenated fats and additives, including sugar it could contain lots of calories. Olive oil, on the other hand has a higher fat content, but is a monounsaturated fat which, if pure, is a natural (good for us in limited quantities) food. Butter, although having a bad reputation may be better for us than margarine, (explanation above) which contains hydrogenated fats. If trying to lose weight, check the fat content *and* the calories.

More Label Reading

Canned and frozen foods may be just as nutritious as fresh but also may have high sodium content. Chemicals are sometimes added to enhance the taste or retard spoilage. Fresh fruits and vegetables may have chemical or pesticide residue so washing them well is prudent.

Highly processed foods may be listed as having the recommended daily dosage of various nutrients but whole foods are in most cases better for us. Plain oatmeal is more healthful than sugar coated oat flakes with added vitamins. Another reason to avoid processed products is that processing components sometimes alter the original foods and may make them less beneficial.

Resource

The FDA Web site can give more information on this subject.

www.cfsan.fda.gov/~dms/foodlab.html

A Sweet by any Other Name

Which is better for us, particularly if we are trying to lose weight? Aspertame®, saccharine, fructose, sorbital, mannitol, or sugar. My nutrition advisor tells me that it makes sense to eliminate the so called "empty calories" of sugar on cereals, in junk foods, cookies and pastries, but she suggests that we do our own research on artificial sweeteners such as Aspertame® and saccharine before consuming large quantities of either. A teaspoon of sugar has no more than 16 calories, which does not make it a big item in a full, daily calorie count but the more we cut out of our diet, the better.

The problem for people who are trying to lose weight comes when sugar is combined with fats in things like ice cream and pastries. A moderate amount of sugar is normally used up by the body immediately and therefore not converted to fat. By eating large quantities of artificially sweetened ice cream in an effort to avoid the sugar, we may be loading on the calories because we haven't cut down on the fat. Cereal with fruit juice is a far better alternative than one with an artificial sweetener but the best is to eat it without any sweetening.

Evaluate New Studies on Food With a Healthy Skepticism

I am like many other consumers who used to respond to every new study like a yo-yo. Some years ago, I remember the worldwide crash of coffee sales when there were allegations that the way it was processed could cause cancer. I believed what I read in the newspapers but found later that the study was badly flawed and untrue. Laboratory animals in most studies are fed huge amounts of substances being tested in an effort to isolate problems. First of all, mice and men are NOT created equal and secondly we probably would never consume the amounts they are given for testing.

It is only as I have done my research for this book both in printed form and on the Internet that I have learned to reserve my judgement until I know where the information came from, who did the study, whether the manufacturer financed it and how it was structured. For now, I figure that moderation in all things is the best approach.

Resource

I found this to be a good layman's guide and easy to understand.
> THE PDR FAMILY GUIDE TO NUTRITION AND HEALTH
> *The Facts to Remember . . . The Claims to Forget*
> *Expert advice on fat, salt, cholesterol, junk food, and your heart*
> *Latest research on stress, cancer, osteoporosis, allergies, and reactions*
> *The medical facts on healing with diet, vitamins, and minerals*
> *Vital tips on energy, fitness, weight loss and gain*

Published by Medical Economics Company—ISBN: 1-56363-135-0
Call 1 800 331-0072 for a copy if you can't find it in your bookstore.

Being Overweight Can Bring Chronic Health Problems at Any Age

Forget the fact that we are constantly exposed to pictures of skinny, beautiful, young men and women leading the good life. We may not aspire to those images even in our dreams but we probably wish we could lose some of the weight that has crept up on us over the years. Many public health experts agree that one of the most serious health problems facing Americans today is obesity. The line between being obese and overweight is not clear but if one is 20 to 30 percent over the average for a specific age and height then he or she can be considered to be obese. In any discussion of maintaining good health and preventing chronic disease, most health experts will stress the necessity of keeping weight within reasonable limits throughout our lifetime. For those of us who missed that piece of advice as young people, it is not too late to enjoy the benefits of a lifestyle change now.

How does one judge whether weight loss is necessary or called for? I have looked at government weight charts and find myself right on target even though I think I weigh too much. I am like many of the people I know . . . I always want to be 10 pounds lighter but from a statistical standpoint, I am not overweight. In other words, a weight that is right for me may be too heavy for you and your particular bone structure. Here are two ways to measure the height/weight ratio.

Finding Body Mass Index (BMI)

BMI uses height and weight to calculate the risk of disease from being overweight.

1. Multiply weight in pounds by 700
2. Divide by height in inches
3. Divide by height again.
4. Round to the nearest whole number.
   BMI under 19 = under weight
   BMI 19 to 25 = a healthy weight
   BMI 26 to 30 = overweight

BMI 31 to 39 = very overweight
BMI 40 and above = Morbidly obese

Another Formula that can be Used

Measure waist while relaxed. Next measure hips where they are largest. Divide waist measurement by hip measurement to get the waist-hip ratio.

1. Ratios above 0.80 for women and 0.95 for men are linked to greater risk for diabetes and heart disease.

The Apple and Pear Comparison

A study done by Harvard Medical School and Boston's Brigham and Women's Hospital, found that a person, who gained 22 pounds or more while an adult, was at greater risk of chronic illness than one who did not.

One expert says that where the extra weight settles is also important. If my profile resembles an apple indicating more weight at the waist and above, I am at increased risk of diabetes, high blood pressure and heart disease. Having a pear shape does not let me off the hook, it still indicates that there is weight to be lost and exercise to be done but is not as strong an indicator of future medical problems.

If overweight for many years, the good results that come from even a modest weight loss and increased exercise could bring immediate benefits, not the least of which is feeling better about oneself.

Exercise—The Best Anti-Aging Medicine There is

I find from many sources that inactivity, both mental and physical is an important factor in functional loss experienced between the ages of 30 and 70. A UC Berkeley Health Newsletter says that one half the age related decline in aerobic power, (how well the heart and lungs bring oxygen to muscles and how efficiently muscles use oxygen to generate energy during sustained exercise), is not due to age but related more to increased body fat and decreased physical activity. Some nursing homes have increased their exercise programs for residents by adding weight training to their therapy. It has been shown to impart many benefits including better balance and more mobility. They have found that even people up to the age of 80 who have lost muscle tone from lack of activity can regain much of what they have lost by a well-planned and directed weight-training program. Another program used with great success with middle aged and elderly people is Tai Chi. Originally taught as a martial art, it is increasingly practiced as a personal discipline that keeps the body flexible, the mind calm and improves one's balance.

Any exercise is better than none.

Five minutes every day of regular exercise is a fine beginning. It gets one in the habit and encourages increasing the time as one gets used to it. A minimum of 30 minutes of vigorous exercise at least three times a week should be a goal.

- A doctor's advice should be sought before starting any strenuous exercise program.
- Don't do too much the first day because it discourages getting out there and trying again.
- Sign up for a program or a personal trainer at a health club or community center
- Exercising in extreme heat or humidity is dangerous for anyone
- Don't call it exercise! Dancing, fast walking, tennis, playing soccer with the dog, biking, and cross-country skiing are only a few. If our goal is to feel better, gain more healthy years and try to cut down on the guilt, it seems clear that limiting weight gain and exercising on a regular basis will "not only add years to our lives, but also life to our years."

How About Trying Weight Training?

People who don't do weight bearing exercise or strength training on a regular basis lose muscle mass every year. Most of us are aware of that. What I didn't know is that we can regain some of that muscle mass if we start a properly planned series of strength training exercises no matter what our age. (We are talking 70s and older) It can help balance, restore a sense of vigor and improve mood as well. No one should walk into a gym and start working out on the big machines without some direction because serious damage can result from unaccustomed exercise but a personal trainer, particularly one qualified to assist the middle aged to elderly person, can tailor a program to one's individual needs and capacity.

Resource

For a copy of this book on exercise call:
Exercise: A Guide from the National Institute on Aging
You can also order a video exercise program for a minimal fee:—800 222-2225—*www.nih.gov/nia*

Dealing with Arthritis—Exercise as Preventive and Pain Reliever

As long as we are talking about exercise, let's talk about arthritis, our nation's number one chronic disease affecting at least 50 percent of persons over the age of 65. This disease has been around since records of civilization have been kept and yet there are still millions of people who experience pain or some degree of discomfort from it. Although there are new medicines coming on the market, traditional methods of treating the disease have not changed. Exercise as therapy is gaining more credibility as practitioners learn how to tailor individual programs to address specific disabilities. I have been diagnosed with osteo-arthritis of the neck, shoulders, hips and knees. Finding ways to stay mobile with a minimum of pain makes a lot of sense to me therefore I am willing to give exercise and/or weight training a try. The possibility now exists to prevent damage to joints through specialized exercise, possible diet changes and treatment with nutrients and drugs. If those treatments can keep discomfort from becoming crippling, joint replacement surgery may become unnecessary. My own search for relief of aching joints has led me on a quest as old as arthritis itself because I am reluctant to take any medication on a regular, long-term basis.

I have been told that appropriate exercise can not only prevent some of the effects of arthritis but also improve already compromised mobility and in most cases relieve pain. Positive results in severe cases may take as long as a year to appear and sometimes one must work through real discomfort to get results. The most important thing to remember is that self-diagnosis and self-training could cause injury and damage to already compromised physical abilities.

Taking Control of the Pain

- See a doctor to identify what is causing discomfort. Osteo-arthritis will require one treatment while rheumatoid arthritis will suggest another but a diagnosis helps to identify that there are no other serious structural deficiencies. In cases of severe joint damage, surgery may be an option.
- Maintain ligaments, muscles, bones and tendons. A key to painless movement of the joints is good health of all the components that are a part of them. Water exercises for those with arthritis offer excellent results in a relatively comfortable, weightless environment as water creates enough resistance to exercise joints painlessly.
- Weight training can be very helpful. Strengthening exercises are important but one should get clearance from the doctor, and advice from a qualified physical therapist or athletic trainer in order to be sure of using the proper technique.
- Walking is beneficial for all parts of the body. Brisk walking,

the use of good athletic shoes and concentrating on having good posture are important for the most beneficial effects.
- Consider diet changes. There are some people who feel that the foods they eat directly affect the health of their joints. It is important to seek the help of a doctor, professional nutritionist, or homeopathic practitioner if wanting to supplement exercise with other therapies.
- Stress has been targeted as a major cause of arthritis pain. Doctors agree that stress aggravates the effects of arthritis and because of that see a relationship between high blood pressure and arthritis pain. Lowering your blood pressure by losing weight, exercising and removing stress from a busy life will also help relieve arthritis symptoms.

Resource

For information on resources the Arthritis Foundation Information Line offers free information on self-help programs, exercise classes and living techniques.—
Tel: 1-800-283-7800

www.arthritis.org

National Arthritis and Musculoskeletal and Skin Diseases Information Clearinghouse—Tel: 1 301 495-4484

www.nih.gov/niams/

This book is an excellent reference for the person who is seeking to improve mobility and find ways to ease discomfort.

ARTHRITIS: WHAT EXERCISES WORK Breakthrough Relief for the Rest of Your Life Even After Drugs and Surgery Have Failed
By Dava Sobel and Arthur C. Klein—St. Martin's Press—1993—
I SBN: 0-312-13025-2

Why Does It Feel So Bad When I Enjoyed Eating it so Much?

Stomach pains, gas, constipation, and acid reflux disease are all covered in excruciating detail on the ads seen during the network news programs. Some of us eat too much of the wrong things too fast and the pharmaceutical companies are stepping up to supply what we need to make us feel better.

People who know about such things say that nothing ages us faster and contributes to more chronic illness and early death than poor nutrition. Add to that a lack of exercise and we begin to understand why the drug companies make so much money responding to the results of poor lifestyle decision-making. Go to any drugstore or supermarket and see how much shelf space is allotted to remedies for digestive problems;

> Acid indigestion—heartburn—Irritable Bowel Syndrome—
> Gas—Diarrhea—Constipation
> Acid reflux—Fiber additives—Stomach soothers—Lactase
> for lactose intolerance sufferers—Enzyme boosters

We Have a Lot of Company

Ronald H. Hoffman, in his book, *Seven Weeks to a Settled Stomach*, says that the National Center for Health Statistics reports that one third to one half of all Americans suffer from chronic abdominal pain. At least 5 million people have ulcers, 6 million have frequent indigestion and 8 million are constipated. Surveys tell us that 18 million people take over the counter remedies for indigestion on a regular basis and 50 million of us take some medication weekly or monthly. As with any problem with one's health, it is important to see the doctor to rule out a more serious disorder.

Some Types of Digestive Problems

Heartburn, acid reflux: Symptoms are pains in the upper chest, neck and back between the shoulders that can sometimes be mistaken for a heart attack. Severe symptoms can include shortness of breath or asthma, hot, burning regurgitation, sore throat and hoarseness. Sometimes called acid reflux disease, it may be caused by improper functioning of the lower esophageal sphincter, (LES), that separates the stomach from the esophagus leading to the mouth thus the contents of the stomach come up the tract instead of going down to the bowel. Gastric acids can then burn the throat.

Course of action: See a doctor immediately if symptoms are severe and to rule out a more serious condition. Eat smaller portions slowly and chew food well. Avoid fried, spicy and highly seasoned foods, fats, coffee, tomato products, and peppermint. One source advises drinking a large glass of water at the first sign of heartburn to flush acidic stomach contents back where they belong and to dilute them. Don't lie down for 3 hours after eating and sleep with a 6 to 10 inch wedge under the pillow or mattress so that the head is higher than the stomach while sleeping. Avoid foods seasoned with monosodium glutamate, (MSG).

Lactose intolerance: This is a condition caused by a deficiency of the digestive enzyme lactase that is responsible for the digestion of lactose, the natural sugar in milk. Not enough lactase means that lactose, found in dairy products, passes into the large intestine undigested where it causes the production of gas and acids that cause flatulence, bloating, diarrhea, cramps, and sometimes constipation. Changes in enzyme production in the body as one ages and sometimes bowel surgery are two reasons this problem may emerge. Some people are born with it, particularly Asians and African Americans.

Course of action: Eliminate dairy foods from the diet for a week to see if the symptoms clear up. Another approach is to ask a doctor to administer a simple test to verify the possibility. This problem is now often called lactose "maldigestion" suggesting that consuming smaller amounts of dairy foods over a longer period of time may ease the symptoms. I don't subscribe to that theory, being lactose intolerant and having tried it to my regret. Since calcium is such an important component of nutrition, not only for teeth and bones but also for the regulation of muscle contraction and relaxation, and blood clotting, women, in particular, need to find some way to keep up their consumption of calcium rich foods. There are pills containing lactase, that can be taken when consuming dairy foods to avoid the adverse effects of this condition and there are milk products on the market that have the lactose removed. Read the labels on processed foods and nutritional supplements carefully because some will contain milk solids causing symptoms to appear in susceptible people.

Gluten intolerance: An intolerance to gluten found in wheat, rye, oats and barley can lead to a condition known as "celiac sprue", which occurs in 1 out of 2500 people, most of whom are women. Symptoms are much the same as for lactose intolerance but include weight loss and fatigue.

Course of action: Cut out all foods containing gluten to see if they are in fact causing a problem. This is a difficult task because many processed foods contain wheat flour: ice cream, salad dressings, canned foods, instant coffee, tea, catsup, mustard and most candy bars. Read food labels and when eating out, always asks the food server for guidance to avoid consuming troublesome foods.

Constipation: The definition of constipation varies widely between individuals. For some, it is infrequency of bowel movements and for others; it is difficulty moving the bowels or movements that are hard and dry. Most doctors will say that a change in what is normal for an individual may be because of poor nutrition, lack of exercise, a side effect of medication being taken, not enough fluids, and even irregular eating habits but the condition should be checked if it persists.

Course of Action: When medication or a structural blockage has been ruled out as a cause, increase consumption of water, fiber, fresh fruits and vegetables. Figs and prunes are great natural laxatives and consuming lots of water plus exercising are important aids to digestion as well. Always have any change in bowel habits checked by a doctor, particularly if there are signs of blood.

Diarrhea: Runny stools, cramping, frequent bowel movements, and thirst are all too familiar symptoms of this condition. Causes can range from disease, incomplete digestion of food, a virus, bacteria found in unfamiliar water, food allergy or intolerance, too spicy foods and/or food poisoning.

Course of action: Replace body fluids with bottled water and nutrients with bland food but if the condition persists or there are bloody stools see a doctor.

Irritable Bowel Syndrome, (IBS): Symptoms include constipation and/or diarrhea, abdominal pain, gas, and bloating.

Course of action: See a doctor to rule out more serious conditions or disease. Since the symptoms are much like those of lactose intolerance it makes good sense to check to be sure that is not what is causing the problem. This condition can be dramatically eased by strict adherence to proper diet as outlined by a doctor or nutritionist and by eliminating stress from one's life.

Gallbladder disorder: The gallbladder is a small reservoir where bile, used for the digestion of fats, is kept. Inflammation of the gallbladder can cause indigestion, nausea or vomiting and fever, which should be treated promptly, as it can be life threatening. Gallstones are small pieces of crystallized cholesterol that can cause intense pain when they become lodged in the bile duct leading to the small intestine.

Course of action: See a doctor immediately. If surgery is not required, it may be suggested that a program of weight reduction be instituted, avoidance of foods such as those containing fats, which can cause discomfort, and change to a low-fat, low-sugar, high-fiber diet.

Digestive disorders caused by side effects from medicine. Possible side affects can range from skin rashes to diarrhea, constipation, nausea and vomiting. Antibiotics, for example, are designed to combat bacterial infections but they don't always discriminate between good bacteria and bad bacteria.

Course of action: Carefully read the literature that comes with medication being taken both over the counter or prescription and follow the pharmacist's directions carefully. A key component of digestion, bacteria also called flora, may be affected by medication and can sometimes be replaced by consuming yogurt with active cultures or acidophilus milk. Some medicines must be taken with food in order to avoid stomach upset. Ask the pharmacist, doctor or nutritionist whether medications being taken could be causing problems.

- A balanced diet, with particular emphasis on fiber from grains, fruits and vegetables, may eliminate many digestive complaints. **Note:** fiber should be increased gradually to avoid over stimulating the system and then kept constant when the right level is found.
- Keep a record of everything consumed in a week if experiencing symptoms of digestive upset. Check it to see if there is any connection between what is eaten and the onset of discomfort. If there is, eliminate that food for two weeks and see if there is any improvement.
- Stress reduction is the key to good digestive health.

Resource

This is a book I found to have clear explanations of problems with digestion and treatment:

>*THE FIRE INSIDE Extinguishing Heartburn and Related Symptoms, Asthma, Chest Pain and Hoarseness.*
>*A Consumer's Guide*
>By M.Michael Wolfe, M.D. and Thomas Nesi—
>New York: W.W. Norton & Co.—1996

I love this book. Not only is it comprehensive, but also it has recipes for foods appropriate to the conditions mentioned.

>*Be Good to Your Gut, Recipes and Tips for People with Digestive Problems*
>By Pat Baird M.A., R.D.—Blackwell Healthcare—1996

Medicine Doesn't Always Make us Well

Self-diagnosis for problems with digestion, the common cold and the flu lend themselves to self-treatment and possibly self-harm. Many of us want the pain and discomfort to go away, NOW and when we find something that works on the symptoms we keep on taking it because we don't want them to recur. Once the immediate problem has been solved, we figure we can look into what must be done to keep us well. Our first line of defense is to see the doctor to rule out the possibility that a serious condition exists. Another consideration is to be sure that drugs taken for chronic illness do not interact with over the counter medications or any natural herbal substances already being taken for other conditions. One drug may alter the action of another by making it stronger thus causing a possible overdose or weaker response therefore losing its effectiveness. Interactions involving alcohol, vitamins, herbals and food supplements can be dangerous to anyone's health. If the doctor has ruled out another problem, making lifestyle changes by perhaps simplifying our lives, reviewing eating habits and easing a stressful schedule could help us more than medication.

A Few Examples of Drug Cause and Effect

- Antacids: Usually prescribed or taken to relieve the symptoms of too much stomach acid, antacids are coming under increasing fire for being useless or worse, harmful. When one takes an antacid for too long the stomach produces more acid in response to the medication thus creating the need for more antacids. Acid plays an important role in overall health by keeping a balance between the beneficial microbes, and bacteria in the stomach that are vital for digestion. It also helps the body absorb calcium and iron. When the stomach becomes too alkaline with the use of antacids, it no longer performs the function of allowing the body to get the proper nutrients from the food eaten.

- Antacids containing **calcium carbonate** sometimes cause constipation. Those containing **sodium bicarbonate** could cause serious kidney problems if consumed with large amounts of calcium from other sources at the same time. **Magnesium hydroxide, as in milk of magnesia** can cause diarrhea. **Aluminum hydroxide** depletes phosphorus in the system and can also be constipating.
- Laxatives: Habitual use of laxatives except the bulk agents can encourage what is known as "lazy bowel" or a dependence on laxatives. **Stimulant or irritant:** These increase the contractions in the bowel. They often contain castor oil, which when overused, can damage the lining of the intestines. **Osmotic:** Causes water to be secreted into the colon. **Stool softeners:** Moistens stool to make it easier to pass. **Bulk agents:** Hold water and make the stool easier to pass. Unless large amounts of water are consumed at the same time they may increase constipation. **Lubricants, mineral oil:** Softens stools so they move through the colon more easily. Too frequent use can interfere with the body's ability to absorb fat-soluble vitamins and nutrients.

Read All the Directions and Warnings on Medications

A study by the General Accounting Office estimated that 17.5% of 30 million Medicare recipients who are not in rest homes or hospitals are being prescribed drugs that are unsafe for their age group. Recent studies have also told us that misuse of medicines such as not taking them as prescribed, not finishing a required dose, taking more than the required number of pills at a time, etc. is behind many illnesses in elderly patients. A large number of them suffer hip fractures each year as the result of falls caused by drowsiness or lack of coordination due to medication. We know that age affects kidney function, which has an effect on the rate medications are eliminated from our bodies. Weight, an increase or decrease in body fat or total body water and muscle tissue can also affect the way the body reacts to drugs. A decrease in cognitive ability could make compliance with instructions for taking a medication difficult if not impossible.

Don't think the elderly are the only ones susceptible. Many of us who are trying alternative medications think they are safer than most prescription drugs but few of us know how they interact with the other substances we put into our bodies. Some herbals can interact with prescription drugs causing serious complications. People of any age can become confused and appear to suffer mental or physical impairment, which can be directly related to the medication they are taking. For instance, antihistamines taken to relieve allergies can cause drowsiness, a condition hazardous to the driver as well as others on the road when driving an automobile. When the label reads that a substance is effective for 12 hours, it means exactly that for most people. I have taken a long-acting antihistamine late in the evening to relieve allergy symptoms while I slept and felt drugged until noon of the next day because I didn't calculate the hour when the effects would wear off.

Don't Fall for "a Pill for Every Ill"

Now that pharmaceutical companies advertise prescription drugs directly to the consumer, the public has been led to believe that they have enough information to suggest and sometimes demand their doctors prescribe something that may not be the best choice for their particular condition. In advertising, companies will describe all the benefits but the risks, as required by law, are mentioned in medical language difficult to understand and print so small one would need a magnifying glass to read it. On television, visual images are designed to sell drugs the same way toothpaste is sold. Cost is never mentioned but can be a vital part of the health equation particularly when the drug being sold is three of four times more expensive than a generic medicine that may work just as well.

Most of us expect a new drug to have been thoroughly tested by the manufacturer and the government. We think we know what risks are involved and whether there is an alternative approach that may be better. The fact is that we don't know unless we have had specialized training and it is the doctor, pharmacist and/or a nutritionist who is our first line of defense in making a decision about whether it is effective and safe. This does not mean that we cannot bring a new drug to our doctor's attention. What we must not lose sight of is that we consult doctors for knowledge, experience and the ability to weigh all the factors necessary to come up with a decision on what is best for us within their sphere of knowledge. To get a complete picture, we should also consult the practitioner necessary to get a better picture of cause and effect of other therapies keeping in mind that herbals and homeopathic remedies could interact with prescriptions and over the counter medications.

Labels of most multiple vitamins and mineral capsules say that they meet the government minimum daily requirements, (RDA), for such nutrients. We should understand that *one compound does not fit all.* Some people need more than that minimum and others less depending on their own body chemistry. Another thing to keep in mind is that not all supplements are readily absorbed by the body. Check the label for the letters USP, which is an assurance that the manufacturer is legally responsible to the Food and Drug Administration for certain standards of disintegration or dissolution, (how fast it breaks up into a digestible mush), potency and purity. An AARP bulletin on being "drug smart" mentions that ethnicity affects the body's reaction to drugs and that a drug rises 40 to 50 percent higher in the bloodstreams of the elderly and lasts 50 percent longer. These are all important facts to keep in mind when we are self-medicating.

The same is true of any medication or drug, the prolonged use of which can cause serious reactions not related to the condition for which it is prescribed. Medicine that was a perfect dosage years ago when it was first prescribed, may in fact be too much for my body to absorb and eliminate properly now that I am older. Symptoms caused by the build up of medications in the system could be mistaken for other serious illnesses, thereby requiring more medications to solve those problems. A recent study indicates that nearly 1 in 20 prescriptions for the elderly are for drugs that should not have been given to them. Those taking medication to reduce the incidence of stroke or heart attack or anti-spasmodic drugs are at particular risk.

Non-steroidal anti-inflammatory drugs, (NSAID), such as aspirin, acetaminophen and ibuprofen, which many of us take without a second thought for arthritis, back pain or headache, can have serious and sometimes deadly side effects. It is widely known that such medications can cause stomach upset and in extreme cases bleeding ulcers. What is not so well known is that some people may have an allergic reaction to aspirin or any medication that contains salicylic acid, the medical name for aspirin. Taking too many too often and for too long a time can cause a rebound effect that will mask the original pain with another. Inappropriate use of Tylenol (acetaminophen) can cause life-threatening damage to the liver if an overdose occurs along with heavy intake of alcohol at the same time. *Read the labels on all medication carefully.* Never combine pain relievers with another over-the-counter medication without checking with the pharmacist to make sure that there is no interaction or possibility of overdosing.

> *A friend of mine was having increasing difficulty with a chronic digestive condition. She tried first one doctor, then another and a third one, receiving a different diagnosis and medication each time only to find that she was becoming more and more ill. She felt she was on a roller coaster as she went from test to test, being told once that it was a terminal condition and another that it required surgery. Finally common sense prevailed and the third doctor took her off all medications, evaluated her diet and lifestyle, and taught her how to deal with stress and the condition eased.*

This is not to say that aspirin or other non-steroidal anti-inflammatory medicines should be avoided. Aspirin has been found to have almost miraculous properties in helping some people maintain a healthy heart but I have relied on my doctor to tell me how a medication can affect normal body function. I also find that in some cases it is easier to ask a pharmacist or nutritionist if I have any questions.

A good plan when a medication is prescribed is to ask that the name, dosage and frequency be written down by the doctor so there will be no confusion. When picking up my prescription, I check that my name is on the container and that the medication and dosage is what I have been told it was to be.

> *One time when suffering from a respiratory illness, I was prescribed a medication by the nurse practitioner to whom I was assigned. I had told both the screening nurse and the practitioner of my allergy to two drugs. Suffering from severe headaches after taking a few doses, I discovered I had received one of those two drugs but had not realized that what I read on the label was another name for one I should not have taken. I did the right thing in telling the first two people treating me of my drug allergies but did not follow through by checking with the pharmacist.*

It isn't enough to know what one's drug allergies are. The same drug may be named two or three different things depending on the manufacturer and whether it is a generic or not. We have to check and double check that what we are taking is what the doctor prescribed, is the right dose and that we know the conditions under which it should be taken. Most pharmacies now provide a printed readout of the information needed to assure oneself of the safety of the medication and some keep a list of the medications one takes so that they will know when a drug is prescribed whether it will interact unfavorably with what is already being taken.

- What are the side effects?
- Does this drug interact unfavorably with other medications being taken? (Including over the counter vitamins, cough and cold medications, etc.)?
- What time of day should it be taken and are there any other

directions that I need to know?
- Should alcohol be avoided? Are there certain foods I should not eat?
- Will it affect my ability to drive?
- Should this medication be refrigerated?

Self-diagnosis and Self-prescribing can be Dangerous

As more and more prescription medications are being sold "over the counter" and thus without benefit of a doctor's oversight, the potential purchaser must take responsibility for seeing that he or she is fully aware of side effects and of individual characteristics affecting what the dosage should be. Some seemingly innocent substances like vitamins, laxatives, antacids, and cold medicines can be lethal if taken improperly or at the same time as other drugs or alcohol. Manufacturers are required by law to furnish information on safe dosage, side effects and conditions under which one should not take specific medications.

READ THE WARNINGS ON THE LABEL OR PACKAGE

Those impossible to read, tiny print instructions on or in the box with medications are there for a reason. I sometimes have to get a magnifying glass to read them or consult a guide to drugs in order to know what I am putting into my body and what effect they could have. Allowing for the fact that each person's body reacts to different substances in different ways helps keep me alert to the side effects of any medications I take, prescriptions or over the counter. Drugs or medications interact with each other, with foods and even nutritional supplements and herbal mixtures therefore I check with the pharmacist, doctor or nutritionist to be sure I am taking them safely.

Note: A drug taken once or twice with no ill effect MAY cause an allergic reaction subsequently.

Resource

I have found this to be informative but useless if not up to date. Look for periodic updates to keep up with new drugs.

The People's Guide to Deadly Drug Interactions
How to Protect Yourself from Life Threatening Drug/Drug, Drug/food, Drug, / Vitamin Combinations
Joe and Theresa Graedon—ISBN 0312 13243-3

There is a very good government site that will give full information on drug interactions, dosage, side effects and precautions for the consumer with links to other interesting Web sites.

www.nlm.nih.gov/medlineplus/druginformation.html

Inventory the Medicine Cabinet

Throw away any medication past its expiration date or that is no longer being taken. Those medicines that weren't finished may have lost their potency. Take time to look at all prescriptions, over the counter medications and diet supplements at least once a year. Check to see how many doctors have prescribed different medications and whether each one knew what the other had prescribed. Then consider how the cough medicines and antihistamines bought over the counter interact with them. Check the resource given above or make an appointment with a nutritionist or pharmacist to check the expiration dates of the medications found on the shelf, interactions from other substances being taken and whether the instructions for taking them are clear.

Resources

Patients can receive free or discounted medications if they meet income requirements and are referred by their physicians. The Cost Containment Research Institute has created a booklet listing phone numbers and addresses of pharmaceutical companies and information on discount mail order services.

Institute Fulfillment Center
Prescription Drug Booklet P—370
PO Box 462
Elmira, NY 14902-0462

www.institute-dc.org

Alcohol. How's a Body to Know?

Most of us are aware that excessive, (3 or more alcoholic beverages a day), and long term heavy drinking may cause damage to brain cells, liver and pancreas and may increase the risk of high blood pressure, or stroke.

Alcohol consumption consumed with some medications, including over the counter types, can cause confusion and diminished brain function, unsteadiness and loss of balance, impaired breathing and stomach bleeding. In addition, the use of alcohol combined with driving can be fatal.

Within the last few years there has been publicity about the possible beneficial results of *moderate* amounts of alcohol. The American Heart Association, The American Cancer Society and the US government have recently issued statements agreeing with that statement. Up until the latter part of 1997, some experts recommended limiting even moderate consumption of alcohol and advocated giving it up completely as it was felt that the incidence of cancer could increase in susceptible people. Recently they revised their stand and said that the risk of cancer in people who consume alcohol is smaller than benefits to a larger population of potential heart disease victims.

One of my friends who is a well-known wine expert tells me that red wine has special beneficial effects because of the grape skins used in the wine making process but a recent study, which received wide publicity said that it did not matter what alcohol was consumed as long as it was a moderate amount and on a frequent basis.

What does Moderate Mean?

Moderation is generally considered no more than one drink a day for women and two drinks for men. A drink is defined as 12 ounces of beer, 4-5 ounces of wine, and 1.5 ounces of 80 proof liquor, all of which have comparable amounts of alcohol. One study implies that people who drink at least that much have a lower overall rate of death than teetotalers, especially from heart disease. As a footnote, it appears that alcohol, such as wine, consumed with food is absorbed more slowly therefore spreading the potential benefits over a longer period of time. In fact, the same amount of alcohol consumed without food loses most of its beneficial effects. What alcohol does, aside from giving pleasure to those who enjoy it, is raise levels of HDL, (the good cholesterol) which helps remove cholesterol build-up from arterial walls and is thought to have other good effects on coronary arteries. Although alcohol is known as a depressant, in moderate amounts it is believed to help people who suffer from chronic stress or depression.

So, What are the Risks?

Alcoholism continues to be a real risk for those people who cannot limit consumption to a moderate amount. Some studies indicate women may be at increased risk of breast cancer because of the effect of alcohol on the production of estrogen but a recent study suggests that a compound found in wine may deter that action. If three times as many women under the age of 75 die of heart disease as breast cancer and 20 times more over the age of 75 then it appears the risk may be worth it. There have been reports that men whose diets are low in folic acid may run a higher risk of colon cancer if drinking any alcohol but increasing the amount of folic acid in the diet lowers that risk. The possibility of increased incidence of osteoporosis in women who drank more than a moderate amount of alcohol had been noted but it is now thought that, in moderation, wine may actually contain estrogen-like substances that could replace some of what is lost naturally after age 50. Regarding the idea that giving up alcohol is a necessary part of losing weight, the American Cancer Society found that moderate drinking caused no weight gain in men and women and in some cases, even some loss.

Note: Men and women, if taking medication for any reason, should be sure there are no harmful effects when drinking an alcoholic beverage.

Now What?

We weigh the evidence, check with our doctor to see if our personal health history indicates we should abstain for some reason, including possible inherited risk factors, do our own research and make up our own minds. Then we should enjoy our beverage of choice, if we wish, with moderation . . . guilt free.

Getting a Good Night's Sleep Can be a Challenge

Sleeping problems often afflict people in their middle years and later. There are many reasons for not being able to get to sleep or for waking before being fully rested; stress, the pain of arthritis, jet lag or change of time zone, a chronic condition, depression, disease, medication being taken for another reason or bad sleeping habits.

Insomnia can be a symptom of a more serious condition such as depression or a primary disorder of its own. It can be transient, short-term or chronic. Not being able to get enough sleep can be a source of stress that in turn makes it harder to fall asleep. In addition to the frustration, one may be less alert during the day thus prone to accidents. Because the immune system can become weakened due to fatigue, one could be more vulnerable to colds and flu.

In other words, we need to do something about it. First, understand that *sleep requirement*, the amount of sleep someone needs, is a very individual characteristic and does not significantly change over the decades of life after the age of 20. The way we feel and whether we can function properly the next day is the best indicator of whether we are getting enough sleep.

From a specialist in sleep disorders, some suggestions

- Check all medications to see if any have a side effect of causing difficulty in getting to sleep or staying asleep.
- Chronic medical conditions such as depression may cause sleeplessness therefore it makes good sense to check with a physician to see if there is an unidentified problem that needs to be treated.
- Focus on the ability to function well during the day instead of how poorly one sleeps at night. A log of the hours we are most alert and able to concentrate on tasks we have set for ourselves is a good reality check. Important meetings or complicated mental activities should be scheduled for those times.
- Bed should be a sleeping place, not a desk for writing letters or for working out intricate problems.
- Establish a bedtime routine that includes applying a hand and body cream that has a pleasant odor just before going to bed. Applying the cream each night is relaxing but it is also a signal to the brain that when it detects that particular smell it is time to go to sleep. (This hint was given in a travel column for people who suffer from jet lag but it has been used as a home remedy for years).
- Maintain a regular sleep cycle by waking up and going to bed at the same time.
- Exercise four to six hours before bedtime. A good fast walk raises body temperature and metabolism. When going to bed, they drop and cause sleepiness. A hot bath or shower can help do the same thing. Although stimulating and increasing alertness at first, two or three hours later both should make one feel relaxed and sleepy.
- Find something quiet to do or read before going to bed that under the best of circumstances can put anyone to sleep; a boring book, a TV program that is not exciting, etc.
- Quiet the mind by writing down important thoughts that

seem to keep one awake. Going to another room and transferring them from mind to paper is effective in relieving worries.

- Avoid bright lights just before bedtime. Use minimal lighting necessary to be able to get around safely and read without straining the eyes. Ambient light, especially bright light, affects the body clock and can delay ability to fall asleep or confuse the full sleep/wake cycle.
- Watch what is eaten and drunk from late afternoon to bedtime. Heavy, fatty, fried and spicy foods may cause digestive upsets that can ruin sleep. The cumulative effects of heavy caffeine use such as in coffee or tea during the day could make one more alert than wanted at bedtime therefore cut back if necessary. Hunger is known in the sleep business as an *alerting mechanism* so try having a warm glass of milk or an herbal tea with some crackers just before going to bed.
- Try drug-free sleep aids available in some drug stores such as adhesive strips, which when placed on the nose, keep airways open.
- Keep hands and feet warm with socks and mittens. It works for me!

Resource

Send a postcard asking for the title and number to AARP;
> *If Only I Could Get a Good Night's Sleep!* A Self-help Guide for
> *Understanding and Overcoming*

Insomnia—
AARP Fulfillment—D 14581
601 E St. NW
Washington, DC 20049

I have checked out this Web site and found it informative and worth consulting for a better understanding of sleep disorders.

www.sleepnet.com

Be wary of over the counter sleep medicines that are antihistamines and can leave one feeling drugged the next day. They also can be habit forming. Each individual's metabolism will dictate how effective they are and for how long they will work. My consultant also tells me to beware of fad sleep aids until they have been thoroughly tested for safety. Dosage of any over the counter sleep aid appropriate for one person may be harmful for another.

> *An 83-year-old man came to see the nutritionist with a complaint of being tired all the time. A thorough history revealed that he had been having difficulty sleeping for many years and his physician had prescribed a commonly used antihistamine for that problem. Often used for the treatment of allergies it has a side effect of causing drowsiness and, taken at night, can encourage a good night's sleep but also can cause sedation and grogginess the next morning. In order to become more alert during the day, he had consumed large amounts of regular, brewed coffee, which kept a high level of caffeine in his system, therefore creating an unnatural balance of waking and sleeping stimuli in his body. Stopping the medication and switching to decaffeinated coffee was all he needed to get a good night's sleep. He learned how lifestyle changes could be successful in helping him sleep and he was alerted to the fact that any medicine taken over an extended period of time should be adjusted to reflect changing weight and age.*

Note: Cutting down on the intake of caffeine should be done by degrees rather than all at once as headaches may occur until the system adjusts.

Snoring May be a Sign of Something Far More Serious than Losing Sleep

We who have suffered from allergies all our lives know that the noises we make in our sleep are less than appealing to our partners.

But for some, snoring may be an indicator that there is a serious condition called sleep apnea causing the problem.

Signs to Look For

- Does the person seem to gasp for air or give loud snorts during sleep?
- Are there long periods when no breathing is detected? How long do they last?
- Does this person fall asleep at inappropriate times during the day?
- Does he or she complain of always being tired?
- Does this person have trouble staying awake while driving during the day?

Sleep apnea syndrome causes a person suffering from such a condition to stop breathing for 10-90 seconds numerous times during a night's sleep. These *apneas*, as the breathing cessations are called, cause brief awakenings. The arousal, sometimes accompanied by a loud snort, is what a body does to "recover" from not breathing. They are so brief they may not be remembered and people affected with this condition are rarely aware that they have been aroused when it occurs. If one suffers many apneas, sleep is fragmented and total sleep is reduced. As a result the person does not awake refreshed and may have to cope with many episodes of sleepiness during the day, including while driving or during lengthy meetings.

Whether we suspect that we or someone else has *sleep apnea syndrome*, it helps to ease the aggravation of our own interrupted sleep if we take time to do a little research by answering the questions above. Aside from affecting someone's behavior by making them tired, irritable and subject to depression, it can cause hypertension and damage to the heart.

There are several treatments for severe *sleep apnea syndrome* that could be suggested by a sleep specialist. Perhaps excess weight should be lost or a breathing machine, (CPAP), which provides continuous positive airway pressure, may be prescribed. The CPAP pumps air into the lungs while one is sleeping so that whenever breathing stops while sleeping, oxygen flow is not interrupted.

For the Relief of Symptoms of Mild Apnea

- Lose weight, if overweight
- Stop smoking
- Don't sleep on your back
- Avoid tranquilizers, sleeping pills and heavy consumption of alcohol. All of these can hinder our body's natural need to keep us breathing.

Resource

This organization supply information on sleep disorders;
American Sleep Disorders Association
1610 14th St NW Suite 300
Rochester, MN 55901
507 287-6008—*www.asda.org*
www.sleepapnea.org

Risk Free Sneezing—
How To Hold Incontinence at Bay

At least 10 million American adults suffer from urinary incontinence at some time in their lives. The problem is more common among women, particularly women over the age of 60 and is one condition leading to institutionalization of the elderly. Approximately one of every five older men has the same problem often associated with problems of the prostate.

It is not only a disorder of the elderly; 10 to 30% of all women are incontinent by their 40's. Excessive weight gain, side effects of some blood pressure medicines, pregnancy, and hormonal or aging changes that slacken the pelvic muscles are all possible causes of incontinence in women.

In many cases reversible, it is more apt to be a symptom of a physical condition that can be treated with behavior modification training, special exercises, surgery or a vaginal hormone cream if it is aggravated by the effects of menopause.

First Step is to go to the Doctor

Get past the embarrassment involved in discussing such an issue with one's doctor. The earlier dealt with the better the long-term outlook is for complete control. There are different types of incontinence but these are the two most common.

Stress, which occurs when one sneezes, coughs, bends, strains, laughs or lifts something heavy, and **urge incontinence** when one must urinate urgently but can't reach a toilet in time.

Non-Surgical Solutions

There are pads or napkins designed for men and women that offer protection and can be purchased at most drugstores and supermarkets. Many people accept this condition, as an inevitable sign of aging therefore don't seek help when something as simple as learning to do exercises on a regular basis could solve the problem. Some women have been advised by their doctors to begin exercises after childbirth and continuing on as a regular daily regimen for the rest of their lives to recondition muscles strained during pregnancy.

The least invasive solution is to do Kegel exercises or bladder training if that is indicated. Kegel exercises are simple to do, once learned and if done regularly can be very effective. Bladder training is a program of scheduled toileting and exercises that help one learn how to control the bladder and is available through physicians or clinics. The bottom line is that those of us who have this problem need to see the doctor to be certain that there are no serious problems causing the condition before proceeding.

Resource

This is a book that could be the answer to an annoying problem for many women and some men. It has very clear and easy to follow instructions to take control of bladder problems. I recommend it highly.
> 7 Steps to Normal Bladder Control
> By Elizabeth Vierck—Harbor Press—1998—ISBN 0-936197-29-3

Incontinence in Men could be a Sign of Prostate Problems

Nighttime voiding, difficulty urinating, frequency, urgency incontinence, and terminal leakage are the predominant symptoms of prostatism. A nagging pain in the lower back, hips or pelvis could be a sign of problems with the prostate and should be checked by a urologist.

Resource

For more information about urinary incontinence contact;
> The National Kidney and Urologic Diseases Information Clearinghouse
> 800 891-5388—*www.nidik.nih.gov.*

For a packet of information on urinary incontinence send a long, self-addressed, stamped envelope and $2 to;
> National Association for Continence, NAFC (MM)
> PO Box 8310
> Spartanburg, SC 29305-8310

www.nafc.org

CHAPTER FOUR

WHEN STAYING HEALTHY DOESN'T WORK

Even when one has made all the right choices and lived life in the most healthful manner possible, illness sometimes catches up with us. How we deal with that reality from diagnosis on will be influenced by the intensity of the will to get well, personality, and the effectiveness of family and friends in supporting us. All of these things supplement the skills of our medical staff.

Stress, a by-product of a hectic lifestyle, plays an important role in chronic illness and the ability of the immune system to fight off assaults from germs, viruses, chemicals in our environment, possibly even genetics or a run of just plain bad luck. A diagnosis of serious illness can create almost unbearable stress of its own so that focusing on anything else may be more than we can muster the energy for. Getting well and the process of healing require that we do what we must to collect the tools needed for that task and learn how to use them in the most efficient manner.

There are several ways to do that and most of them require becoming actively involved in the management of one's own illness and treatment. Our modern healthcare demands that we take more personal responsibility for our own healing and recovery. It is hard work to be an active participant in the decisions we are sometimes called upon to make, but it is better than trusting to luck and being a passive victim of circumstance. Sharing our concerns, questions, confusion and even low spirits . . . talking to others who have suffered from the same condition . . . helping someone else find solutions, learning new approaches to treatment, giving and receiving comfort; all of these are active attempts to understand and give a manageable form to a serious illness.

Having someone act as an advocate, supporter, spokesman and guide in assessing the complicated choices with which we may be faced is a gift beyond counting. From speaking to people who have been through traumatic illness, I have learned how quickly life can spin out of control before one finds the strength to move from one decision to the next, from one painful treatment to another and another. Sometimes we need all the help we can get.

Battling Chronic and Serious Illness

Kenneth R. Pelletier in his book, *Sound Mind, Sound Body: A New Model for Lifelong Health* writes of a five-year study showing that good health in many cases is related to attitude. He refers to it as an "inner quality" that gives rise to coping strategies in response to life's hard knocks. The people he refers to who have successfully dealt with serious illness, viewed each new trauma as a challenge and committed themselves to finding a solution rather than denying that it existed. He identifies the key to recovery as the effort to exert some control over tough circumstances rather than having a hopeless or helpless attitude. The most skilled doctors in the world and the most advanced medicines cannot make us well if we are unable to focus our energy on what it takes to fight being discouraged.

At this age, I find more contemporaries facing chronic or serious illness than at any time previously. I interviewed a friend as she was recovering from surgery for a malignant tumor in her breast. She shared with me her shock when the diagnosis was made, how she became overwhelmed by her feelings of confusion, fear, and even anger as her peaceful life suddenly took on a wholly different set of priorities. At the same time she was concerned for how her husband would deal with her illness, the possibility that surgery and recovery would make her feel less attractive, less than a full-time partner in their marriage. Others mention that their life has an unreal quality to it, as if they were seeing it in a movie. I find from my research that these feelings are not unusual. Those who have recovered speak of the necessity of regaining the energy lost that comes from all those emotions and of struggling to turn it into a powerful force for recovery. They learned everything they could about their illness, asked questions, and never gave up their search for the best doctor or treatment until they found the right match. Creating a sense of purpose beyond an overwhelming preoccupation with the diagnosis made them begin to get a grip on the new reality of their lives.

Why we Need to Get Smart in a Hurry

Treatment options can be complex with pluses and minuses for each one. Some doctors are more skilled than others, some are able to communicate better than others, one medical center may be more experienced in treating a specific condition than another, and often there is no absolutely clear choice for what course should be followed. In some cases, momentous decisions must be made based only on what feels right and the trust placed in the doctor.

When it involves our own health, we have to do more than hope that our doctor is the wisest and most qualified. His or her experience and skill are what we rely on to properly evaluate and treat an illness. It would seem that if we are being asked to make important life choices, we should know how to evaluate the doctor treating us, to weigh the options available and then learn what it takes to become a skilled team player in fighting for our health.

RESOURCES

Have not had occasion to use these Websites myself but they could make a diagnosis of serious illness a little clearer, calculate the risks involved of various treatments thus helping to make the decisions necessary in a life and death situation.

    American Cancer Society—*www.cancer.org*
    American Lung Association—*www.lungusa.org*
    American Heart Association—*www.americanheart.org*
    Mayo Clinic—*www.mayoclinic.com*

Sometimes We have to Go with our Instincts

A friend told me of suffering increasing pain for months thinking that it was a minor injury resulting from a fall. Finally she went to a doctor who wanted to do a diagnostic procedure that her HMO denied because of the cost. He did not indicate that it was a matter of life and death and thus she was not alarmed. It was months later when the pain had become unbearable that she went to another doctor through another health system and a malignant tumor was discovered.

Suspecting that something is seriously wrong and not feeling comfortable with the diagnosis that has been given, gives us the right and mandate to keep pushing until we get an answer we are satisfied with. Time can be an important factor in the treatment of some illnesses so we can't afford to jeopardize our chances of recovery with indecision.

Resource

This book makes good reading even for someone who is not ill. Aside from the honest retelling of a tortuous journey, the courage shown as the author pulled himself from the despair of an "inoperable" brain tumor and the clarity with which he describes his lessons learned make this well worth reading. It is full of important lessons if one should ever become seriously ill.

Making Miracles Happen—By Gregory White Smith and Steven Naifeh
A New York Times Notable Book—1998—ISBN 0-440-50837-1

For support/education groups helping people who have chronic or life-threatening disease;
The Center for Mind Body Medicine—1 202 966-7338
www.cmbm.org

For information on other approaches to cancer treatment
The National Foundation for Alternative Medicine—1 202 463-4900—
www.nfam.org

The Communication Age is Here. But Use it Wisely

If higher survival rates from serious illness are associated with a sense of coping or a feeling of being in control then educating oneself is the place to start. Such efforts take enormous energy and perseverance but the value of getting insights into our illness so that we can know the questions to ask our doctors is beyond measure. The library is a great place to start. Since most of them have computers, the Internet as a source of information is available. If one is not comfortable with computers, the references needed, lists of national organizations representing the condition being researched, and lists of support groups in the area can all be found in the local library.

The Internet:
Is it a Treasure Trove or a Misleading Waste of Time?

It is a lot of both. If, during the course of an illness we are required to weigh several options, none of them absolutely guaranteed to be successful, knowledge helps decision making become a more orderly process. When everything works well, the Internet can be an invaluable tool but at its worst, it can be dangerously inaccurate and misleading. No one becomes an instant expert by consulting the Internet but being more knowledgeable about an illness, perhaps being able to bring information on a new treatment to the doctor's attention might make a big difference in one's recovery. Talking with others who are experiencing the same pain or frustrations could bring important insights into one's own attempts to cope. A doctor must stay current with fast moving advances in his own specialty that may include hundreds of diseases and problems while carrying a full load of other responsibilities. As patients, we have the luxury of concentrating on our own condition but unless we have a trained medical background, we lack the knowledge and experience to tell us what to reject and what to value.

Not every patient has the sophistication to evaluate the huge amount of information now available nor is every doctor open-minded enough to accept that a knowledgeable patient is a patient who has the energy and will to get better. The fact remains that we will receive better medical care if we know more about what ails us. Our responsibility is to show the doctor that we can sift relevant information from sensational and poorly researched, out of date material, and that we know how to cross-reference what we find.

Because anyone can access medical information on TV, newspapers, magazines and the Internet, more patients are willing to question their doctor's decisions. A patient with a serious illness can no longer trust blindly that the doctor assigned, the hospital where he or she has privileges and the staff working there are the best to be found for that patient's particular condition.

As mentioned before, the consumer is being forced to become proactive in managing illness, treatment and recovery by finding the most effective and best health care possible. It is as important to any strategy for recovery as the treatment chosen and the Internet is one of the easiest ways to get smart in a hurry.

Why Many Doctors are Less than Pleased with all this New Knowledge

- Some doctors worry that their patients will become needlessly depressed over their prognosis from what they read in magazines, newspaper articles or on the Internet.
- Some are offended when they feel patients are questioning their knowledge. They suspect that some people don't know as much as they think they do.
- Another complaint is that it takes valuable time from the business at hand to counter incorrect conclusions found on the Internet.
- Conversely, there are doctors who feel that it makes explanations easier and saves time if the patient has some knowledge of the illness.
- Many doctors consult the Internet also but have more experience in evaluating what they find.

Important Things to Remember

- Never substitute advice found on the Internet for a face-to-face with the doctor.
- Regard every study or discussion on the Internet or other media with a healthy dose of skepticism. Understand that information found on the Internet may not be accurate. Statistics can be manipulated to reflect the writer's point of view. Some studies are structured better than others and some may be outdated. We must rely on common sense and instinct to help us select what is valuable.
- The Internet is only one tool among many that can help in a search for recovery and healing.

Questions to Ask Oneself

- Has the study appeared anywhere else? The Journal of the American Medical Association, New England Journal of

Medicine, Lancet and other prestigious medical publications should be referenced.
- Was it peer reviewed?
- Did it involve human or animal studies? If animal, for instance, then the results are only indications that they may be useful for humans.
- How timely is the information and when was it last updated?

Not All Web Sites are Created Equal

Check out the Web site selected to see what credentials are listed for the writer. Some researchers at Ohio State University found that even the most prestigious university sites contained inaccurate and incomplete information because the creators of the Web site rarely consulted their own doctors and researchers about the content. Government sites tend to be ultra-conservative and commercial ones push their own products or treatments.

Some Web sites on health matters are assessed for accuracy, timeliness and content, but because there are others added to cyberspace every day, it doesn't hurt to keep looking. It is suggested that until there is a better review process, users should rely on information from trusted peer-reviewed sources. The safest way to be sure of information is to cross-reference anything we find by using standard medical texts and periodicals.

RESOURCE

Although this Website is mentioned in other areas of the book, it is particularly pertinent when discussing using the Internet in order to research any serious illness. Find the Website and then go to:

How to Evaluate Health Information on the Internet: Questions and Answers—
www.cancer.gov

Support groups found in "chat rooms" on the Internet can be very comforting. Several people have mentioned the benefit of sharing information with others suffering from the same illness this way, especially those run by national patient support organizations. Aside from talking with those who are going through the same things, success stories and effective treatments found by others may end up saving a life. Moral support, found by talking with sympathetic individuals, is an integral part of treatment and recovery both for the patient and for loved ones.

- Save time by learning the mechanics of search engines: If typing in "cancer" using any of the most popular search engines, one might get over 14 million matches, as they are called. Narrowing the search by entering a specific cancer and you could get 1 million. After being as specific as I can, and when I have found what I need, I make note of where the information was found or use my Internet program's bookmark system to be able to return whenever I wish.
- Before sharing information from the Internet or any other source with the doctor, see whose Website it is, the date of the articles in it, and whether a government, university or commercial organization has sponsored it. No doctor will diagnose or treat a patient based on information from sources not known or trusted and that includes the Internet.
- Most doctors do not want to diagnose or suggest medication for anyone by email. Check to see if short communications, such as questions on prescribed treatment or medication could be helpful on Email but don't be surprised if the doctor would rather conduct business on the phone or in person.

Resource

For many health related questions this is one of the most informative and well-presented Websites.—*www.mayo.edu*

One of the most up-beat and informative presentations of how to take control of one's medical care and, in this case rehabilitation for physical disability is the following that is published as a joint venture of the National Rehabilitation Hospital Center for Health & Disability Research, The Medstar Research Institute and funded by Paralyzed Veterans of America and Eastern Paralyzed Veterans Association, Inc.—Tel: 202 466-1900

The Keys to Managed Care: A Guide for People with Physical Disabilities—

www.nrhchdr.org

www.pva.org

www.epva.org

Here is a Website that gets high marks on accuracy and timeliness. It is easy to navigate and provides links to many other Websites of interest.

www.healthfinder.gov

If you are one of those who wish to take advantage of these resources but do not use a computer, ask someone who does to print out the information for you or go to your local library and ask the librarian for assistance

---

Becoming an Active Member of the Team

Managed care has forced many patients to change the way they interact with their doctors. Some people feel that they are rushed during appointments and don't have the time to ask all the questions they want or even to develop a personal, trusting relationship. When one has been diagnosed with a serious illness it could be a key to recovery. In interviews with people who have found this to be true, some have adopted ways to make the most of the time spent with the doctor. They start by sorting out their goals and priorities.

- Does the doctor listen to me and take an active interest in what I say?
- Can I tell him what he needs to know to treat me effectively?
- How much do I really want to know about my condition?
- If the treatment is arduous with the possibility of limited success, is quality of life more important to me than prolonging it?

- Do I have the energy and will to pursue the suggested courses or treatments? How much risk am I willing to accept?
- Have I the willpower to make lifestyle changes if there was hope of turning a serious situation around?
- Would I be willing to accept surgery as an option? What odds of success am I willing to accept if I decide to have surgery? Am I willing to do the research necessary to see if there are alternatives?
- In considering chemotherapy or radiation, how do I feel about the possibility of pain or changes in my appearance?
- Does my medical insurance cover the costs of treatment or is there a possibility that I cannot afford the proposed treatment?
- Is my age a factor in how much the doctor or I am willing to do to recover my health?

Once I know the answers to these questions, my doctor can assess, not only my willingness to become a proactive member of the health team treating me but also what course of treatment best fits my own personal wishes. It is in this way that we can begin to move from being a victim of circumstances into regaining some control of our lives.

Ways to Get the Best Value From Your Doctor's Visit

- Find the best doctor. I feel that the definition of a good doctor is one who is compassionate in the use of exceptional skills and will be there when I need him or her. This is especially true if one is elderly. A doctor may be more aggressive in treating a younger person but willing to give up on someone who is older. Word of mouth helps in the selection process and is a good indicator of competence and caring.
- Get someone else to sit in on doctor's visits. Two heads are definitely better than one in such situations. It is difficult for a patient to keep track of complex decisions to be made

or procedures being proposed under the best of conditions but when traumatized by a serious diagnosis, it is even harder. Questions that should be asked may occur to a companion more readily and the answers might help all concerned. A tape recorder could do the same thing if the doctor does not object.

- Form a partnership with the doctor. Patients I have interviewed said that they made it clear they wished to be involved in decision making, that they wanted their questions answered in a way they could understand, and that they wished to feel as though their opinions were valued. Liking the doctor as a person is important because we need a good working relationship. Keep in mind that a good "bedside manner" is not necessarily an indicator of skill. It just makes one think so. Communicating well is a vital part of the recovery process. If there are problems, find another doctor.
- Developing mutual respect means that one is mindful of the doctor's need for the patient to be clear and concise about his or her condition. At the same time we want to feel that we are getting the very best care available. The doctor's training, his or her success rate and experience are important parts of one's decision making particularly if surgery is being proposed.
- Trusting the doctor means that once we have made a choice we will keep an open mind about his or her suggestions for treatment. This does not mean that everything should be accepted on blind faith. It implies that if the doctor brings us along by explaining each step in the process we will direct our own efforts to complement his. There is a certain time when trust in the doctor's wisdom and one's own instinct will hopefully give us confidence and peace in our decision making.
- Being realistic does not mean that one has to give up hope but it helps some people to know what the odds are and what weapons they can bring to bear on the problem.

- Ask for a second opinion if feeling uncomfortable with a recommendation made by the doctor. It's *our* body and *our* life.
- Ask what the doctor is hoping to achieve with a proposed treatment.
    Will it prolong life? Are we talking 6 months or 6 years?
    Is the treatment an extra insurance against recurrence?
    Will it minimize the pain although not prolong life?
    What is the quality of life I can expect while undergoing treatment and after?

- Keep a daily health log between visits to the doctor while being treated. It is difficult to keep track of all the questions to ask about things like appetite changes, new aches and pains, or the side effects of newly prescribed drugs.
- Share responsibility for the recovery process by doing what the doctor asks. Get instructions in written form during appointments so the details won't be forgotten. If medication is to be taken for a certain number of days, finish it unless told otherwise even though one feels better before then. Willingness to comply with suggestions to lose weight, give up smoking or exercise regularly, are a direct reflection of how much one is willing to do to get well.
- Mistakes could be hazardous to our health; Keep in mind that anyone, doctor, nurse, pharmacist or technician, even the best, can make mistakes. We must be active, alert and assertive partners in the delivery of our health care to keep those mistakes from causing serious problems.
- If one is referred to a specialist, ask for information about that person in order to encourage confidence in his or her ability to treat the condition successfully. Again, if the doctor is working with an HMO, the choice of specialists may be limited so we must evaluate the person to whom we have been assigned and know how to seek another if we are uncomfortable with that choice.

Resource

It is possible to check to see if a physician is board-certified in his or her specialty on the Internet.

American Board of Medical Specialties' site—*www.certifieddoctor.org*
American Medical Association, Physician Select—*www.ama-assn.org*

Prepare a Summary Before you Go

There was an article I read, which gave what I think is valuable advice for the process of being proactive about getting the best medical care we can. We know that the time a doctor can spend with us is limited so we want him to have every piece of information he needs to be able to evaluate our personal medical profile. A way to do that is to go through the medical file we will be taking with us and put all the information the doctor could use in diagnosing the problems we present on a "cover sheet". It could save duplicate tests, could raise a flag if there are genetic considerations and prevent adverse drug reactions. This piece of paper could then be your "crib" sheet in filling out the usual medical history forms when arriving at the doctor's office.

- Record all pertinent insurance information including membership or ID numbers and contact information for the insurance companies.
- List all medications being taken, how often, how much and when. (That includes over-the-counter pills, herbal or homeopathic compounds and supplements)
- Informing the doctor of all known drug allergies is absolutely vital.
- List every condition for which one is being treated presently, for how long and the name and phone number of the doctor being seen.

- Regularly scheduled medical tests such as mammography, prostate, colonoscopy and the dates they were administered are other items to include.
- Past history of treatment for other conditions is also important information so list what they were, the dates and whether hospitalization or surgery was required.
- Family history is an indicator of possible genetic conditions of which the doctor should be aware.

Why a Second Opinion Could Save Your Life

When given a bad-news diagnosis requiring a difficult procedure or surgery must be performed, one wants to go to the best, most skilled doctor in that field. Usually a patient is referred to a surgeon or specialist whom the primary doctor is associated with, is in the same medical group or perhaps has a good reputation for that type of surgery or condition. Sometimes the name comes from a list of surgeons in a specialty provided by your insurance company. For many of us impatient to get the surgery done or treatment started right away, worried about perhaps offending our doctor, or waiting to make another appointment, getting that second opinion does not have much appeal. The fact is that although not a great many decisions will be reversed by doing it, if a misdiagnosis is found in one's case, it could be the best time we ever spent.

Getting a second opinion, once we have been told what the diagnosis and suggested procedure is to be, is a way to insure that not only is the diagnosis correct but also that the treatment plan is the best one. An article I read recently says that one in five second opinions result in a different diagnosis or if not, can produce an alternative treatment plan. If you are not satisfied with either diagnosis or there is a major difference in opinion, ask your insurance company if they will go for a third opinion to be used as a tiebreaker. When the diagnosis is based on lab reports from a biopsy, a second look at that biopsy by another pathologist is good insurance. Mistakes have been made on reading the results and biopsy samples have been mixed up in the lab leading to misdiagnosis. Make sure, when going for a second opinion that the lab reports are being reviewed. Remember also that practicing medicine is a skill and an art. Some are better at what they do than others. Your challenge is to find the doctor with the most experience and the highest success rate.

> *A friend was diagnosed with prostate cancer. He had an appointment with one surgeon who informed him that the procedure would require damaging nerve bundles thus leaving him impotent and incontinent. He decided to see if he could better his prognosis by going to another doctor skilled in this area, which he did and has recovered completely from his operation.*

Most HMO's or managed care plans usually pay for a second opinion but patients should call to find out exactly what will be covered when going for one. Medicare will also pay the costs for a second opinion where surgery, radiation or chemotherapy is recommended. It is also good to know that laws in 42 states and the District of Columbia back up a patient who wishes to have an independent review of their HMO or medical plan's treatment decision.

What Everyone Should Know About Heart Disease

I did an informal survey of women friends recently, asking them what illness they most feared and all but one mentioned breast cancer first. A few listed heart disease as a concern. No one mentioned stroke as a cause of death and each of them said that they dreaded the possibility of Alzheimer's disease. Many studies indicate that heart disease is the leading cause of death for American women.

Although women have fewer heart attacks than men before menopause, the risk grows to be almost equal to that of men afterward and more women die of cardiovascular disease than do men. The theory is that higher levels of the good cholesterol (HDL) that are linked to the maintenance of a healthy heart are associated with the production of estrogen. After menopause as estrogen levels decrease, the production of HDL also decreases. Statistics from several studies imply that 940,000 people 250,000 of them women, die of heart disease every year and that, within those numbers, Hispanics and African-Americans have multiple risk factors for heart disease.

Genetic factors may predispose one to heart disease, so if there is a family history of such problems, it would make good sense to know what needs to be done to stay healthy. The first and most obvious is to talk to one's doctor to find out what our risk factors are and decide what lifestyle changes we must make in order to lower the chance of a heart attack.

What Numbers We want to See on our Blood Tests

Learn how to read blood test results and know what the figures are for LDL, (the bad guys), HDL, (the good guys), and Triglycerides as well as total blood cholesterol. The National Cholesterol Education Program says this is what one should hope for;

- A blood cholesterol level of less than 200 milligrams/deciliter
- LDL of less than 130 milligrams/deciliter
- HDL of more than 40 milligrams/deciliter for men, 50 milligrams/deciliter for women
- A ratio of 2.5 or lower (The ratio is found by dividing the total blood cholesterol level by the HDL figure)
- Triglyceride level of less than 200 deciliter

Some Strategies for a Healthy Heart

- Pay special attention to diet.
- Keep blood pressure within normal limits. High blood pressure is the number three cause of fatal heart attacks.

- Avoid smoking.
- Exercise, exercise, exercise!
- Learn how to deal with stress. Easier said than done but taking courses such as yoga, meditation or stress management could help.
- Know what the symptoms of heart disease are.

   1. Chest pain that comes and goes or tightness that moves into the jaw, left arm, shoulders or neck
   2. Chronic breathlessness, especially at night
   3. Overwhelming and unusual fatigue
   4. Dizziness, lightheadedness, fainting, sweating and nausea
   5. Swelling in ankles and legs

Resource

This website is really interesting, easy to use, and informative. It is an independent educational Website with information and services for prevention, diagnosis and treatment of cardiovascular disease.

Heart Information Network

www.heartinfo.org

Would I Recognize a Stroke or Brain Attack if I were Having One?

Most of us know the symptoms of a heart attack but if we experienced random nausea, dizziness or numbing of one side or temporary vision changes we would probably blame the flu. Not recognizing what could be a serious problem or reacting quickly enough could impair our ability to recover from such an event if it were indeed a stroke. If there is an emergency facility which has a stroke protocol, speedy diagnosis and possibly treatment with a blood clot dissolving drug, tissue-plasminogen activator, (TPA), administered within three hours of onset could make a dramatic difference in recovery.

Stroke or brain attack is one of the most costly diseases in the US today due to expensive and lengthy rehabilitation required of those who do not die from their attack and the need for care incurred because of disabilities limiting mobility. The cost in human terms of losing function once taken for granted is enormous.

Using figures given in a newsletter from our local hospital center, approximately 500,000 to 700,000 people suffer one or more strokes yearly. Of those, 150,000 die within a year. As one ages, the risk of brain attack grows and if one is male or African-American, even more so. A family history of stroke can increase the risk. TIA's or transient ischemic attacks, can strike silently and frequently enough to cause increasing cognitive loss leading to possible misdiagnosis of Alzheimer's disease. Almost 25 % of those suffering such TIA's will have another stroke within two years.

It is important that all of us know what the symptoms are and then get help from an appropriate emergency facility if there is a suspicion that we are suffering an attack. Being mistaken is quickly forgiven. It is better to be safe than sorry.

- Know what the symptoms of TIA's and major brain attacks (strokes) are.
- Difficulty speaking—Double vision, blurring, loss of vision—Sudden severe headache
- Dizziness, unsteadiness, sudden falls—Unexplained nausea, vomiting—Sudden weakness or numbness of the face arm or leg on one side of the body
- When having a physical, ask the doctor to assess the risk of a stroke or brain attack. High blood pressure is a significant indicator of the possibility of stroke. Heart disease can result in breakaway blood clots, another major cause of stroke. Diabetes increases risk because of damage to blood vessels in the brain. Cigarette smoking, high alcohol and drug consumption are also risk activities. Some prescription medications have a side effect of raising the possibility of stroke.

- If a stroke is suspected, call an ambulance. Time is critical and paramedics can alert the hospital to be prepared for a possible stroke victim so diagnosis and treatment can begin immediately on arrival.
- If someone we know is at high risk of stroke ask them to find out from the doctor what nearby hospitals have stroke protocols and can administer TPA therapy after determining the type of stroke that has occurred. Damage could result from TPA therapy being used for the wrong type of stroke.

Resource

These organizations offer information and resources for stroke survivors and caregivers.

The National Stroke Association—Stroke Connection—96 Inverness Dr., East, Ste.1—Englewood, CO 80112-5112

www.stroke.org

American Heart Association—7272 Greenville Ave.—Dallas, TX 75231—Tel: 800 553-6321

www.americanheart.org

NINDS Neurology Information Office—P.O. Box 5801—Bethesda, MD 20824

www.ninds.nih.gov

Guess what . . . Men Get Breast Cancer Too!

Having known two men in the last year who were diagnosed with breast cancer, I thought we women should become as informed about the possibility of the men we care about getting breast cancer as we are about our own chances. We should encourage everyone, male and female over the age of 40, to perform self-examination for lumps in the breast but also to have any suspicious discoveries checked by a doctor.

The American Cancer Society Web site on men's breast cancer emphasizes the same early detection proviso as for women and although the risk for men is rare, the possibility of not considering an unexplained lump in the breast as being cancer is higher with men for obvious reasons. Most of the publicity we see is about women's breast cancer but because men have so much less breast tissue, a small lump could spread to other tissue more readily if not detected early.

The National Cancer Institute has devised a Breast Cancer Risk Assessment Tool that could change the way women, particularly those over the age of 50 view their chances of having breast cancer sometime in the future. It is based on data from 250,000 women and can be accessed through the National Cancer Institute. Although breast self-exams are still a good idea, research has indicated that regular mammograms and in some cases ultrasound examination are the most effective ways to detect early breast cancer.

Obviously, each of us needs to bring to the doctor's attention any genetic predisposition to breast cancer. One's present age, the age at which menstruation started and when our first baby was born are also important indicators. The average age when breast cancer is diagnosed is 63. Hispanics and Asians have lower rates than Caucasians but African Americans are more likely to die of breast cancer than whites.

Early diagnosis of breast cancer and treatment with new drugs continues to give hope of increased survival rates from this disease. As with any disease, the more we know about it the better able we are to make proper decisions and focus our energies on getting well.

Resource

I found these organizations to be very helpful and the Web sites easy to understand.

The Cancer Information Service—800 422-6237—*www.nci.nih.gov*

American Institute for Cancer Research Nutrition Hotline—800 843-8114—*www.aicr.org*

American Cancer Society 24 hour info-line—800 227-2345—*www.cancer.org*

This site provides information on the side effects of cancer treatment, has an oncology nurse to answer questions from patients and caregivers 24 hours, and assists with coping strategies for chemotherapy induced anemia.

The Oncology Nursing Society—*www.cancerfatigue.org*

This organization helps women learn how to feel beautiful again after cancer treatments.

Look Good . . . . Feel Better—800 395-LOOK

The Association of Cancer Online Resources (ACOR offers access to 131 mailing lists that provide support, information, and community to everyone affected by cancer and related disorders.—*www.acor.org*

What Every Man and Woman Should Know About Prostate Cancer

Prostate cancer is the most commonly diagnosed cancer in older men, affecting one in eleven. It is usually found in men 65 and older and in half of all men over the age of 80 in the US.

In its early and curable stages, the disease rarely causes symptoms. Concurrent problems, such as benign enlargement of the gland can cause difficulty with urination and irritative symptoms such as frequency, urgency and nighttime voiding. A digital rectal examination (DRE) and a blood test, (PSA) are recommended yearly commencing at age 50 or earlier if there is a history of the disease in one's immediate family or if one is an African American.

There are many factors to be considered in the treatment of prostate cancer, among them one's age, whether or not the disease is limited to the prostate or has spread, the rate of growth (Gleason Score) and the PSA level. The earlier the disease is detected the more treatment options will be available and of course, the greater chance of cure.

- Insist on a yearly prostate examination. Persistent symptoms such as difficulty urinating, burning, frequency and urgency, cloudy urine and bleeding, even if transitory should be warnings that seeing a physician is demanded. Denying that recurring and annoying symptoms could be an indication of something far more serious is not unusual. Since there are few middle-aged women who have not suffered a urinary infection at one time in their lives, recognizing the symptoms of urinary distress in someone else should not be difficult.
- Do what it takes to become informed about prostate cancer. There are many options for treatment of this disease so deciding on a course of action is difficult. A diagnosis of serious disease is difficult enough but prostate cancer and its treatment involves our deepest feelings about each other and brings up matters we may not be used to talking about together such as the possibility of impotence or incontinence. These complications will vary with the form of treatment and should be discussed in detail with one's physician.
- Understand that within the medical profession there is not universal consensus at this time on the best course for detection and treatment of prostate cancer. Some patients opt for surgery and others for watchful waiting. One doctor might suggest radical surgery where another may not. Many people struggle with weighing whether the risks of incontinence or impotence are higher than the possible benefits of treatment. Look for several opinions from recognized authorities in the field, and ask friends who have already been through diagnosis and treatment for their advice.
- As with any serious illness, find the most successful treatment center. Do research and listen to recommendations of others.
- Join a support group to help relieve the worry, frustration and fear. If you use the Internet, search for as much information as possible and share concerns with others who

have "been down the same path before" by signing on to "chat rooms" found through well-recognized groups.

Resource

Sponsored by the American Cancer Society, this book helps one through the emotionally trying quest for the best options for treatment.

Informed Decisions: The Complete Book of Cancer Diagnosis, Treatment and Recovery
By Lois B. Morris and Dianne Lange—American Cancer Society—2001—ISBN 0944235271

Alternative or Complimentary Medicine and Integrative Therapies

Dr. James Gordon, in his book, *Manifesto for a New Medicine,* relates his experiences trying to get relief from pain resulting from a back injury using the traditional methods of Western or allopathic medicine with which most of us are familiar. Told by his colleagues that there was nothing more they could do for him and being unable to function due to the pain, he pushed himself to move beyond the boundaries of traditional medicine for relief.

In desperation he consulted a doctor who used what might be called in this country nontraditional healing arts. After a complete and pain free recovery he changed the way he looked at medicine forever. As Director of the Center for Mind-Body Medicine in Washington, D.C., he is, in his own words "working to create a more compassionate, open-minded and effective model of health care and health education" that he refers to as the *New Medicine* and specializes in the care of cancer patients.

Conventional medicine has been enormously successful in treating overwhelming infection, surgical and medical emergencies. Gene therapy is also showing great promise but chronic conditions such as hypertension, arthritis, multiple sclerosis, asthma, and cancer among others are still causing immeasurable misery at great expense. Powerful medications may cure the symptoms of one condition but damage other systems and organs within the body. "Super bugs" are proving resistant to antibiotics that were once so successful in dealing with bacterial infections. Long-term use and abuse of steroids by athletes to increase muscle strength and performance, and by people suffering from chronic pain have been found to result in sometimes fatal and often seriously debilitating conditions. Non-steroidal anti-inflammatory medicines used indiscriminately for chronic conditions such as arthritis can bring on serious stomach problems and do nothing to improve the underlying cause of the disease.

More important from Dr. Gordon's point of view is that health care providers no longer have the time to find out about the whole person when trying to bring someone back to health. Patients, in his words, "want and deserve someone who will listen respectfully to us, who will take seriously our point of view about the problems that are deforming our lives, who will help us help ourselves." He feels the patient of today is more willing to take responsibility for self-care and self-knowledge than he or she has been given credit for heretofore.

He also points out that many alternative methods of medical treatment, aside from being successful in treating chronic illnesses, are less costly than many present traditional treatments and procedures.

Resource

I found this book moved me from skepticism to cautious willingness to pursue alternative and integrative medicine as described by a traditionally trained physician.

MANIFESTO FOR A NEW MEDICINE, Your Guide to Healing Partnerships and the Wise Use of Alternative Therapies
By James S. Gordon, M.D.—Addison—Wesley Publishing Co., Inc.—
ISBN 0-201-45383-1

Dr. Gordon's center publishes a newsletter I found very helpful in providing resources for those searching for alternative treatments for cancer as well as giving an understanding of how traditional medicine can be integrated with such treatments.

The Mind-Body Connection—Published quarterly—202 966-7338

How to Find the Most Effective Treatment

At this writing there are over 200 alternative therapies available to the medical consumer in this country. Andrew Weil, a well-known author and expert on alternative healing methods, feels that all of them are mixtures of wisdom and foolishness. He maintains that western trained physicians who are familiar with alternative forms of treatment are better able to detect conditions that could be treated by traditional western procedures while at the same time being able to advise on the benefits of other treatments. That makes good sense to me.

I am not alone in wanting to have the best of both worlds. Americans spend large amounts out of their own pockets for what some used to call "breakaway treatments" but are reluctant to abandon the medicine they know. HMOs, insurance companies, supermarkets, pharmacies, health food stores and medical practices are beginning to respond to this desire for more effective treatment of chronic illness. They are beginning to see the cost benefits of offering greater access to alternative therapies and medicines. The production of vitamins and other food supplements is a multi-billion dollar business in this country and rising all the time.

Resource

Operated by the National Institutes of Health experienced information specialists can answer questions about federally funded research into alternative medicine and will send packets on current research being monitored by the Office of Alternative Medicine Clearing House.

Call Monday through Friday, 8:30AM to 5PM Eastern Time—
888 644-6226—*www.nccam.nih.gov*

Found a very informative Website called Alternative Health News Online that is up-dated daily and provides links to other interesting sites.—www.altmedicine.com

In response to increasing demand some clinics or medical practices provide services that take a holistic approach to their patients. Rather than treating symptoms of a specific disorder, they treat the person as a unique individual with special qualities and problems that need a customized treatment approach. Time is taken to understand all the factors of a person's life and to evaluate the effect they may have on total health.

Resource

For information on holistic medicine as well as ways to find a practitioner;
Holistic Medicine Web Page—www.holisticmed.com
The author, trained in traditional Western medicine and thoroughly educated in alternative therapies has books, newsletters and "healing tapes" available for those who want more information on shaping a health policy for themselves. His books are easy to read and understand for the layman.
SPONTANEOUS HEALING How to Discover and Enhance Your Body's Natural Ability to Maintain and Heal Itself
By Andrew Weil, M.D.—Published by Ballantine Books—1996—
ISBN: 0-449-91064-4

These are Some of the Therapies.

Acupressure is the application of fingers on special points to relieve stress, pain and spasm.

Acupuncture is a technique that was developed in China over thousands of years ago. Needles are used to stimulate points on the channels of vital energy or Qi (pronounced "chee")

that flow through the body, and influence the balance of the body's natural health. It is used to relieve chronic pain and specific maladies such as migraine headaches.

Aromatherapy uses inhaled or rubbed on scents to change behavior and mood. They are also used to treat some diseases.

Biofeedback helps one to learn how to regulate and control stress-related physiological and mental processes by interpreting signals from the body.

Body/mind medicine deals with mental and emotional influences on physical health. Reducing stress through meditation, yoga, guided visualizations, biofeedback, positive thinking and body-oriented psychotherapy are some of the methods of treatment used to great success on the theory that stress worsens virtually every illness.

Chiropractic therapy use physical force to manipulate the spine to treat muscular and skeletal disorders. The theory is that spinal problems can interfere with nerve supply and blood circulation to the rest of the body and are therefore responsible for pain and disease. By treating such problems, chiropractic therapy can therefore benefit general health.

Conventional Western medicine as we know it is oriented toward symptom relief, the control of infection and surgical solutions to physical ailments.

Herbal medicine often practiced by naturopaths, treats disorders with medicines that are derived exclusively from natural plant materials. Combining long-standing insights into health and healing with modern pharmacological research, it is practiced widely in Europe and the Far East. Remedies that are specifically suited to each person's individual needs are prescribed in order to help the body heal itself. It is used as a self-help system of health care, and professional interest in it is growing. Chinese herbs are sometimes prescribed as a supplement to acupuncture treatment.

Holistic medicine is the practice of considering the whole person in treating disorders rather than treating individual symptoms.

Homeopathy is a holistic approach to healing based on the principle that "like cures like" and that symptoms of illness are expressions of disharmony within the whole person. It is a system of medicine that stimulates the body's own natural defenses and curative powers. Homeopathic medicines are administered in extremely diluted form and work by influencing the "vital force" or energetic level of the body. Perhaps the most important characteristic of the homeopathic practitioner is the skill of listening to the patient and evaluating all the factors in that person's life before recommending a treatment.

Naturopathy emphasizes restoring good health or wellness to the whole person through natural means. Dietary modification, vitamins, extracted food supplements and extracts of whole leaves and barks are important in treatment.

Osteopathy, like chiropractic therapy, uses manipulative techniques to adjust structural misalignments of the body. Because nerves from the spinal cord supply the whole body, the theory is that spinal problems are often related to other disorders. In most parts of the US, osteopathy is practiced as part of standard Western medicine. The physical technique is often referred to as osteopathic manipulative therapy.

Spiritual healing includes many faiths, Christian Science, Faith Healing, Healing ministries, Native American spirituality, and Scientology among others and concentrates elements of faith and prayer on the healing process.

Therapeutic touch therapy and massage are used to stimulate healing by improving circulation and for the relief of acute and chronic pain. There are many types; neuromuscular therapy, muscle energy manipulation, Swedish, myofascial release and Rolfing are some. Shiatsu and acupressure, as practiced by highly trained specialists, shares many of the same principles of acupuncture.

Resource

This is considered a definitive guide to alternative therapies. It got a very good review in Cooking Light Magazine.
Alternative Medicine: The Definitive Guide, Second Edition
By Burton Goldberg—Ten Speed Press 2002—ISBN 1587611414

Are All Alternative Therapies, Food Supplements, Vitamins and Herbs Safe?

As with any medicine or treatment, side effects, the implications of long-term treatment, and the efficacy of each approach should be investigated. Just because something is natural or a friend has been taking it for years does not mean that it is entirely safe for someone else to take. Herbs taken at the same time as some prescription or over the counter drugs can cause serious problems. A licensed practitioner, pharmacist or doctor should be consulted on combining them. Look for the word "standardized" on the label to ascertain strength of the primary ingredient. Some herbs are known to cause serious liver problems and others can raise heart rate as well as blood pressure.

If it is true that each body is unique it follows that one person may be sensitive to a substance where someone else is not. At the moment, there are few regulatory standards or established safety criteria for substances such as medicinal herbs classed as food supplements. There is no guarantee that the herbal or the dose suggested is effective or safe so we must know and understand the effects of any substance or therapy we undertake for our health. We have to do our own research to find the brand name or supplier with the best reputation. A nutritionist knowledgeable about herbal medicine as well as pharmaceuticals is also a good source for information.

Resource

The National Center for Complementary and Alternative Medicine provides information on its Web site, which I found to be very easy to navigate and also relatively up-to-date.—*www.ncaam.nih.gov*

I like this book for its reasoned and realistic approach to alternative therapies and medicines. It gives a clear picture of what should be known before embracing any treatment.

THE ALTERNATIVE MEDICINE SOURCEBOOK. A Realistic Evaluation Of Alternative Healing Methods With Information on: The strengths and weaknesses of alternative approaches, Finding a qualified practitioner, Integrating conventional and alternative medicine, Recommendations for common illnesses
By Steven Bratman, M.D.—RGA Publishing Group 1999—ISBN 1-56565-626-1

Rosenfeld's Guide to Alternative Medicine. What Works, What Doesn't and What's Right
Dr. Isadore Rosenfeld—Fawcett Books 1998—ISBN 0-44900-74-5

If The Doctor Recommends Surgery

We have all read horrifying stories of the wrong leg being amputated, friends who have come home from the hospital fighting a stubborn infection picked up in the hospital or the effects of an adverse reaction to anesthesia or medications. There is no question that mistakes happen; Harvard made a study of 30,000 hospital charts and found that nearly 3% of patients were injured by some preventable mistake. In some hospitals the average is higher and if we are included in the 3% that is too high a risk. An Institute of Medicine report says that 44,000 to 98,000 people die in hospitals each year from medical errors. No matter whether you think the numbers are inaccurate or seem high, if you don't wish to be a statistic you have to become an activist on your own behalf and minimize the risks.

- Information about the surgeon chosen for one's surgery particularly how often he or she has performed this type of surgery, the success and complications rate and how others knowledgeable in that particular discipline feel about this surgeon's skill are key components to the decision making process. Find out if the surgeon teaches at a hospital or a medical school thereby increasing the chances that he or she has kept up with all the latest developments in this specialty. And by all means check to see if the hospital where the surgery is to be performed has a satisfactory rating from the proper regulatory agency.
- Question proposed preoperative tests. There is no reason to run up costs or to be put through additional discomfort by having unnecessary tests but keep in mind that some doctors may prefer to have their own hospital lab do the tests. If they have been done within one month, ask why they have to be repeated. Be aware of all the risks involved, as some tests can be hazardous to one's health. Read carefully the waiver of responsibility if required to sign before some procedures
- For elective surgery, most hospitals will bank one's blood for transfusion on the day of surgery, if necessary.
- Find out which doctor will have primary responsibility for the post-operative care as we probably won't see much of the surgeon who did the surgery once we get back to the room. Know the name of the resident who will be directing daily care and the interns who will be following up with routine care and what their duties will be. This helps keep one's expectations in line with what really happens.
- Ask the doctor if antibiotics are to be administered before the operation to help fight post-operative infection and then check with the nursing staff to see that it is done the

prescribed length of time before surgery. This is especially important for the outpatient surgery patient.

- Be aware that consuming food or drink twelve hours or less before general anesthesia is administered can cause devastating effects during and immediately after surgery. Don't assume that all staff and visitors know a surgical patient must fast before surgery. Refuse any food or drink mistakenly offered or the surgery could be postponed at the last moment. Much surgery is done on an outpatient basis so the patient must take responsibility for following directions on the consumption of food and drink.
- Ask the doctor what is planned for pain control ahead of time. Pain and related stress can slow recovery and increases the risk of complications. There is some evidence that certain relaxation techniques and stress reducing exercises such as yoga and biofeedback done before surgery will greatly reduce anxiety and tension therefore lowering the level of pain afterwards. See if the hospital offers such services. Some procedures respond to patient-controlled intravenous analgesia, (pain medication), a system allowing one to control and relieve pain by pushing a button on a computerized pump.

> *A friend regaining consciousness from surgery on her spine, was told that she was to use a morphine pump to control pain particularly as the surgeon wanted her to remain still to allow the extensive incision to heal. As her pain became unbearable, her husband suspected that the machine was defective. When receiving no response from the medical staff, he asked how it worked, watched it carefully and took notes. Armed with that information, he went to them and proved that it was not doing what it was supposed to do. Pain is a relative thing and hard to judge when it is not one's own. The staff thought that since the machine was expected to work properly his wife was experiencing discomfort rather than severe pain. It was her husband's persistence and insistence that moved them to replace the defective*

pump with another one bringing her some measure of relief. Having her husband stand in and stand up for her was invaluable to her recovery.

Someone recovering at home from outpatient surgery was given pain medication and to relieve the resulting nausea was given a common anti-nausea medicine. Within a few days of taking it, she experienced severe headache, pain and stiffening in the jaw and swelling of her tongue. Not having been told that such a reaction could occur from the anti-nausea medicine, she went to the local emergency room to be given a dose of an antihistamine and the symptoms disappeared. She should have been made aware that such a reaction could occur but it would have been better if she had double checked herself.

- Once the doctor has done his part, the patient shares responsibility for his or her own recovery. Deep breathing exercises are sometimes prescribed after surgery in order to help clear the lungs and reduce the risk of pneumonia. If surgery is planned, ask if there is any benefit to these exercises before surgery. Ask if doing the Kegel exercises before prostate surgery could make recovery from incontinence after the operation speedier.
- After many procedures, getting on one's feet as soon as possible may seem cruel and unusual punishment but it also may be vital to making all systems begin to work again. It can prevent phlebitis, which is the formation of dangerous blood clots resulting from lying in bed for long periods of time, and cut down on the risk of pneumonia.
- Be the first line of defense in avoiding serious drug interactions and problems. Bring to the hospital a list of the drugs, vitamin supplements and over the counter medications presently being taken so they can continue to be given in the hospital if it is permitted. Ask the doctor to write a list of the medications to be given in the hospital; name, dosage, purpose and if possible, get a description of color and shape. Use that list to check medications each

time they are brought and ask the doctor to review the list every 72 hours. The identification wristband given on admittance to most hospitals should list drug allergies and sensitivities. Ask the nursing staff to check it each time they bring medication, particularly if a change is noted in what has been received before. Check the IV each time it is started and renewed to be sure it is the correct one. If eating and drinking normally, one may not need to continue IV treatment.

- Ask the doctor to leave standing orders to treat two common post-surgery problems, constipation and insomnia if necessary.
- Know what tests the doctor has ordered while in the hospital. Ask whether they are really necessary or could be postponed.
- Keep a pen and pad of paper handy to write down questions to ask the doctor when daily rounds are made. I am a great believer in keeping a journal. Reading it over can give insights into one's own strategy for recovery and it helps chronicle thoughts during a very stressful time.
- Be a pest. Ask questions. They could save your life.

All of this pre-supposes that one will be in a condition to pursue these initiatives but if not, a family member, relative or person holding the health care proxy can ask them. A list of these questions written before surgery will give that person an idea of your concerns.

Resource

I have scanned this and although never admitted to a hospital except for births of our two children, found it could be very useful.
HOW TO GET OUT OF THE HOSPITAL ALIVE: A Guide to Patient Power
By Sheldon P. Blau and Elanine Fantle Shimberg—Macmillan, New York—ISBN 0-7858-120-91

How to be an Effective Medical Advocate

The partner and/or family members of someone going through hospitalization for serious illness or surgery often struggle with their own feelings of distress and helplessness. They try to find the best formula to be a support and comfort while not intruding on the patient's need for privacy. Some choose to become an advocate for those who because of their illness or incapacity cannot be one for themselves.

> *The husband of a friend of ours became her advocate, advisor, cheerleader, mentor and constant well of support in the hospital when she had two cancer surgeries. Drawn by a unique relationship to share the trauma his wife was going through in the most meaningful manner possible, he used his professional training as an aviator and senior naval officer to evaluate the effectiveness of every aspect of her treatment. He helped her make decisions when she could not make them and constantly bolstered her will to live when she couldn't think why she wanted to. He was in on every conference with the doctors, researched every aspect of her disease and when he heard of a new treatment he conferred with her doctors and put them in touch with the people who could advise them. He talked to friends who might be able to give him other leads. He participated in the vital monitoring of her immune system, the ups and downs of red and white blood cells as she went through chemotherapy by creating graphs for himself so that he could recognize changes before they became serious. They both speak of the cooperation and commitment of her doctors and all the medical staff to making her well but it was his familiarity with the details of her treatment that made him a valid participant in the team approach to her recovery.*

Not everyone has the skills to be as involved as he was but there are things we can do for someone for whom we hold a Health Care Proxy. To be a really effective advocate for a seriously ill patient, we should be aware of the commitment of time required and the emotional investment of such a mission.

What an Advocate Can Do

- Don't let anyone treat a lingering condition in a routine manner. Denial and delay could change the odds of recovery.
- Teach yourself to be completely objective. It is important to hear and record everything then let the patient decide what decision to make based on the facts. If you tend to retain only positive or negative information ask to hand off the job to someone who is not so emotionally involved.
- If a second opinion is called for, suggest going to a doctor in another institution and that new tests be done to double-check the first ones.
- Correct diagnosis is the first key to recovery. If there is uncertainty with a diagnosis, insist on further tests even if insurance will not cover them.
- Be clear on what the patient's wishes are. Ask if the Living Will and Health Care Proxy are legal in the state where the patient is. Talk over what expectations the patient has on quality of life issues and how much friends and relatives should be told about his or her condition. We need to know how involved the patient wants an advocate to be.
- If accompanying the patient to doctor's appointments before surgery, take notes so that what was said can be reviewed at a quieter time. Help the person write questions down before going to the appointment and ask those questions for him or her if the need arises. If something is confusing, ask for clarification because it is likely the patient did not understand it either.
- Surgery and hospital stays require skills of observation and willingness to ask questions. When a patient advocate is dealing with someone else's life, it is important to be assertive but not combative in a way that could help the staff detect mistakes in the administration of medicines or treatment.

The fact that someone else is watching for these things reassures the patient that he or she can concentrate on recovery alone. Because the people treating us don't want mistakes to happen either, they will hopefully appreciate another set of eyes and ears to help them.

> *A friend had an operation on the spine near the anal area. Everyone was aware that the risk of infection was high and life threatening. Her advocate made sure he knew what time her dressings would be changed each day and was there to be sure that strict attention to sterile techniques were followed. No one knows if he saved her life, but the fact is that the nursing staff knew he was there to see that they followed procedure and she did not suffer a subsequent infection.*

- Win the hearts and minds of nursing and medical staff. Do what it takes to be aware of the awesome responsibility they hold in the recovery of your patient. Remember that on night duty and holidays they forego being with their own families to care for your patient and others. Pursue issues with vigor if necessary when questions arise but avoid confrontation and seek opportunities to praise extra effort or kindness. Remember . . . unless we have had medical training in their particular specialty, we may be way out of our field and need as much help as we can get.

Dealing with Serious or Terminal Illness

Diagnosis of a serious illness may be so shattering that it can leave one emotionally and mentally paralyzed. I read an article recently in AARP Magazine that I thought was one of the best outlines on what to do after getting such bad news that I have seen. I have added some items that I consider important as well.

- Once the diagnosis has been made, put together your own strategic "strike" team. This should include the best doctor

for your particular condition, and a medical advocate, (see above).
- Appoint an information disseminator, to field phone calls and inquiries from concerned friends. You can also put an up-dating message on your answering machine and screen calls as they come in.
- The preceeding means that you have made a decision as to how much you wish to share with your friends.

> *A friend recently went through successful treatment for breast cancer. She chose to share her diagnosis and subsequent emotional ups and downs with friends. Her openness and quest for information created a bond of caring and concern that helped with decision making and buoyed her during the dark days. People who had been through the same experience gave invaluable advice on everything from side effects of radiation and ways to ameliorate them to treatment options and how to evaluate them. She controlled the information but she gave us the signals we needed to give her the support she wanted.*

- Unless a good case can be made for immediate action, don't let anyone rush you into a decision before being able to evaluate all your options.
- Although your primary care doctor may have seen you through many traumatic incidents, he or she may not be the most qualified person to oversee your condition and treatment. Making the right decision on who is to have your life in his or her hands may be the most important one you make.
- I have mentioned this before, but it doesn't hurt to reinforce it. By all means get a second opinion and even a third if you can. (Not in the same practice because the likelihood of contradicting one another is not high)
- Devise a strategy to have your doctor listen to you but stick to the important details. He is as anxious to have you be informed as you are to know what is going on.

- Become a sponge for information on your illness. (Check other sections and resources on the subject in this book)
- If your condition calls for a stay in the hospital, choose it as carefully as you would your doctor.

Resource

For medical information to help one make informed decisions about treatment or health care being proposed, consult this source. Library personnel will tailor their search to each person's case and provide the best scientific information available.

The Stanford University Medical Center's Health Library—800 295-5177
www.http://healthlibrary.stanford.edu

To get a quick overview of your hospital's ratings try this Web site.—*www.healthgrades.com*

We had a close friend who was fighting a serious illness and for some reason went into a coma from which the doctors had little hope of rescuing her. For three weeks she fought off the crises and finally emerged weakened but also very aware of some of the things that had been going on around her. Her family was key to her recovery and the subsequent struggle to regain her mental acuity as she recovered. The daughter gave me some interesting insights on things they did to help themselves help her that I share with you. The intensive care unit nurses gave them an understanding of what was going on but family members used their instincts to devise strategies on their own.

- Nobody speaks in absolutes and can't be expected to. This is probably the single most difficult thing to understand when trying to get a handle on what's happening and what may happen tomorrow.
- Often the staff will tell what not to do but not explain what can be done to give comfort or express concern especially if

the patient is comatose. Always ask. Their experience could give valuable clues to what could be done. They did tell our friend that her mother could sense her presence although not acknowledge it.
- Operate on instinct. If the person loved music, try playing a favorite tape now and then. This friend used to read poetry to her mother and it helped her learn to ignore the machines and beeps and tubes.
- Attach "Post-it" notes to the chart for questions to ask the doctor with your phone numbers they can easily reach you.
- Respect the professionalism of the staff. The nurses carry a huge amount of responsibility and stress. Our job is to be a comfort to our patient and theirs is to care for that person without interference.

When Coming Out of Surgery, Coma or Serious Medical Episode

- Expect confusion. Do not be surprised if it takes weeks to bring someone who has been unconscious for a long period of time back to full cognition.
- Allow the patient to focus on one thing at a time. My friend brought several personal mementos; a photograph of a happy moment, a child's drawing or a shell picked up in the summer to help bring back memory. The patient may not be able to contribute much but it is a way to get thought processes going again. As her mother recovered, an album of photographs from home of a trip they had taken together gave them something to help bring back memories.
- Bring a small treat to eat when recovery is on the way. A Big Mac may not sound like a big deal to you and me, but when you have been in the hospital near death, it may be just the ticket. (Of course, check to see if it is allowed on the patient's diet)
- Write down the experiences the patient relates. It may be difficult to recognize them as reality but in this case the patient wanted to work her own way through what was very real to her.

- Remember that a seriously ill patient is often self-absorbed and has no energy for anything but recovery. Part of your gift to this person is not to expect a callback or even a thank you when notes and gifts have been sent.

Decoding, Demystifying and Surviving the Medical Bills

Anyone who has been involved with our present system of medical care knows just how frustrating and confusing it is to receive a hospital bill or deal with charges for prescription medication. With a hospital bill, understanding what each of thousands of entries are, whether they are accurately listed, how much will be paid for by insurance or how much by Medicare is a daunting task. Hospital billing offices do make mistakes and sometimes very costly ones. If skilled in this area, by all means follow the labyrinth, question the billing by doctors, laboratories or hospitals and when feeling as though one is being treated unfairly explain, clarify and persist in fighting for a review of the bill and perhaps an adjustment. Not only is it unfair to the consumer but also to Medicare to be billed for more than they should be required to pay. Basically, I feel as though I am the first line of defense in trying to keep medical care fraud and mistake costs down because I feel we all end up paying in higher insurance premiums.

A friend sent me the following account of trying to help her mother receive the prescription benefits that she felt her insurance policy provided for.

> *"In 1999 my 85-year-old mother was diagnosed with Parkinson's disease. Her doctor prescribed a brand name drug and specified that he did not want her to be given a generic substitute. It was her understanding that her Medicare supplemental health insurance policy included a prescription benefit providing that she co-pay $5 for each 30 day supply. When I picked up her medicine, her insurance company declined to pay the $80 cost. Directed by the pharmacist to contact her former employer for a clarification of the prescription benefit of*

her group supplemental medical insurance, the employer was unable to produce a list of specific benefits and directed me to the insurer. The insurer said no statement of benefits was available and sent me back to her employer. Because my doctor husband told me that it was illegal to withhold a specific statement of benefits to the insured, I called the insurer a second time to inform the representative that the company was bound by law to produce the statement. I gave my mother's name, ID Number and address. Because of a number of events in our lives, nothing more was done until Spring of 2001 when I was told, after repeated phone calls, that a statement of benefits would be mailed to my mother. It arrived in December 2001 and confirmed our memory that for each 30-day supply of medication her policy required a $5 co-pay. Armed with this statement and her insurance ID card, the pharmacist was told by the insurer that her mother would need a letter of "medical necessity" from her doctor to receive a prescription benefit for a brand name drug. A letter of "medical necessity" was faxed from the neurologist to the insurer and the benefit was finally allowed. In an attempt to file a claim for compensation for the 2 years that she had to pay full price for the medicine, we were told that she could only claim for one calendar year from the date of the filing of the claim. 3 weeks later, having not received the form, I called again to find that they had no record of the request but would mail a form that day. A month later when none had arrived, I called once again to tell that representative that I had made a note of her name, the date and time of my call and the next call would be from my mother's attorney. The form arrived 4 days later. Now the fight begins to get full compensation for the elapsed time from the first denial of benefits to the admission of coverage.

If the battle is too complicated and time consuming my suggestion is to hire an expert to fight it. There is so much we don't know about our rights and benefits and so much insurance companies and hospitals have to gain by counting on our not knowing that we need to help ourselves become better educated. I am not implying that they are actively trying to cheat us; just that billing has become so complex that even they do not always know where the arbitrary rulings and double billings impinge on our rights. See below for how to find someone who can help.

Resource

I haven't reviewed this book but the title leads me to believe it could be helpful. It is a guide to understanding what your policy benefits and exclusions are, and how you can identify mistakes and rectify them.

>*Making Them Pay*
>By Rhonda Orin—St. Martin's Press—ISBN 0-312-2670-6

In looking for the most comprehensive website on the subject of money management for the average consumer, I found the following. It had a full explanation of what a daily money manager does and how to find one in one's local community. To order the complete Aging Parents and Adult Children Together, A/PACT series:

>Consumer Response Center
>A/PACT: Daily Money Management Programs
>Federal Trade Commission
>Washington, DC 20580—toll free: 877 382-4357

This group can supply a list of names of daily money managers in one's own community.

>American Association of Daily Money Managers
>PO Box 755
>Silver Spring, MD 20918—301 593-5462

Medical Billing Advocates of America can give you the name of a local affiliate who will check your hospital bill for overcharges and underpayments by your insurance company. As this book goes to print, they are about to bring out a workbook to help amateurs like me do the same thing.—540 387-5870—
>*www.billadvocates.com*

A Medical Profile Could Save Your Life in an Emergency

Think through the details of facing an emergency situation. Chronic medical conditions sometimes require specific treatments; some of us are allergic to certain medications; any one of us might require a transfusion of blood but valuable time could be lost while medical personnel try to find out what blood type we have. Medical staff making decisions about one's care in an emergency could be saved vital time if they had specific information about an individual's health facts. In cases of non-life threatening injury, hospitals are reluctant to treat patients if there is no proof of ability to pay. Knowing my insurance company and account number could speed things up considerably. Notification to my family in an emergency could be made in a timely fashion if the hospital had a name and telephone number at hand.

An Emergency Health Care Packet, with all the information medical personnel would need could be compiled and left in a handy place near the front door. It should be kept up to date as medications are added or dropped and someone other than us should know where it is. (See Appendix B)

Many of us drive or fly long distances, far from the familiar territory of our own doctors and friends who know us. Suppose I decide to go skydiving in Chile and am taken to a medical facility to repair the damage? Doctors could find information about my health profile invaluable. A laminated Emergency Health Care Card carried in the wallet with the necessary medical facts on it can be quickly referenced if needed. (See Appendix B)

CHAPTER FIVE

RECOVERY, HEALING AND CAREGIVING

As I have mentioned before, fast-moving events can change lives. An automobile accident, diagnosis and treatment for catastrophic or chronic illness, or being sent home from the hospital before being fully able to take care of oneself means we might need some help. Independent life can be transformed into total care in a matter of hours at any age. For the elderly who are living alone, gradual loss of cognitive function or decreasing mobility may cause relatives and friends to worry that assistance is needed to ease a difficult living situation. For others, the daily tasks associated with independent living such as shopping for and preparing meals, bathing, dressing and getting in and out of bed could be temporary problems needing some assistance or they could be indication of a slowly deteriorating lifestyle.

Finding the right combination of care, tailoring it to one's own needs or trying to help someone else requires using skills for which most of us are unprepared. My husband and I have been in such a position three times and have learned much about what works and what doesn't. If I were to point out the three most difficult problems, the solutions to which bring the greatest rewards, it would be to

- Evaluate the level of care required accurately.
- Have someone accept the help offered.
- Find a care giving solution that "fits" with the patient. This includes in the hospital, rehabilitation unit, nursing home, one's own home or wherever the recovery or care is to take place. Having to check and recheck that arrangements negotiated and arranged for live up to the expectations of both the patient and caregiver can be frustrating.

Concentrating on Healing and Recovery After a Hospital Stay

Recovering from surgery or fighting chronic illness calls for resources from deep within, a willingness to follow the doctor's instructions and the ability to focus energies on what it takes to recover health.

- Be on the lookout for signs of infection. Ask the doctor or visiting nurse about any condition that indicates recovery is not proceeding properly. Wash hands frequently or use "towellettes" and remind caregivers to wash their hands before any personal contact.
- Encourage relationships that are conducive to feeling peaceful and happy. Don't worry about hurting feelings if some friends are not helpful to the process, it's more important to save your energy for getting well.
- Therapies such as bio-feed back training, yoga and spiritual healing can be used to create a quiet state of mind and body to encourage a good response to treatments. Look into other methods of healing that could complement traditional treatment, give peace of mind, and control stress. Some patients have found that it reduces the need for pain

medication. One friend gave a gift of massage to someone struggling with rehabilitation from a stroke. Another friend going through chemotherapy received a gift of a make-up and makeover session when the effects of treatment made her feel less than beautiful.
- Seek professional help if the illness and resultant stress cause family relationships to suffer. Recognize that both patient and caregiver or partner will at some time grieve for what used to be. Discouragement, fatigue and frustration are normal, but self-defeating thoughts need to be dealt with. Acknowledging all of these feelings, finding a way to solve problems and then moving on are signs of recovery.
- Set priorities. There are many activities we crowd into a day that are habit rather than necessity. Doing the things we enjoy is important to recovery. Those other things can be saved for when we are well.
- Encourage a sense of humor. The mind and body work together to recover from illness and it helps those suffering through trauma to enjoy a light moment now and then.

Caring for Someone Else . . . a Cram Course in Planning for Oneself

Many of those aged 50, 60 or 70 are in a unique position. Hopefully healthy, and energetic they are, in many cases, pursuing full time careers or perhaps retiring and shifting to less demanding occupations. Since many couples are marrying later in life, they may still be raising children at the same time as their parents are showing signs of needing help. Sometimes quite suddenly due to illness, an accident or a phone call from a concerned neighbor, they find themselves stepping in to assist a parent who, from earliest memories, had been self-sufficient. Welcome to the "Sandwich Generation". As a result of my experience in caring for elderly relatives, many friends have consulted me about their parents or relatives whose problems are becoming *their* problems. They all expressed surprise that they found themselves in this position.

My husband was still on active duty when my 84-year-old mother was diagnosed with a terminal illness. The most acute memory of the following 4 months is how abruptly life changed for her and for me from the moment we left the doctor's office. We were so numbed by the implications of her illness and subsequent surgery that it was difficult to discuss financial issues with her when we were preoccupied with medical decisions. She had a Living Will because we insisted on it but we knew nothing of a Durable Health Care Proxy or Power of Attorney, and luckily it was not required at that time. Once she returned home from the hospital, juggling daily requirements of two households, hers and ours, was often exhausting. My sister was able to move in with her to supervise her care, otherwise it would have been much more difficult. With no experience in providing 24-hour care, little knowledge of how she wished to receive that care or whether she had the resources to pay for it, my siblings and I trusted to instinct and often hearsay advice to keep her comfortable. It was a time fraught with uncertainties and mistakes, but we succeeded in providing for her comfort until the very end.

For those of us who have faced this dilemma, lessons learned include wishing we had known more about home health care, what needs to be done to safeguard against theft, improper care and physical or emotional abuse by the caregiver who has been entrusted with a loved one's care. (See Managing a Home Health Care System) We would like to have been more confident that there were enough financial resources to pay for the care being given and to know how we could find more if they were needed.

Watch with Patience and Listen with Wisdom

The need to remain independent, the desire to manage on one's own, a reluctance to be a worry to children or friends, causes many people to deny both to themselves and others that there is anything wrong. Some people can successfully mask a growing inability to manage daily needs like paying bills, getting in and out of the shower or driving a car until a crisis makes it obvious.

For Someone Living Alone the Slide Downhill Can Go Unnoticed

- Declining eyesight makes driving difficult to impossible as well as dangerous.
- Not being able to drive to get groceries means having to ask others for rides.
- Difficulty getting groceries means increasingly poor nutrition thus lower resistance and immunity to illness.
- Not eating well can cause depression, mental confusion and symptoms mimicking dementia.

Determining when problems have escalated into the need for intervention requires more than tact. It means being knowledgeable about the inter-relatedness of nutrition to depression and depression to physical health. We need to be aware that not all doctors know how age affects the absorption and elimination of medications from an elderly person's body therefore risking the devastating effects of over-medication. We have seen that even when the change in lifestyle is gradual, the willingness to project thoughts to the possibility of someday needing assistance ourselves becomes more difficult as we get closer to it.

I have a friend who has retired from his own very successful career. His father, a man in his 80's, had been parent, role model, advisor and authority figure, was living by himself and seemed to be having difficulty managing his financial affairs. It was discovered that a door-to-door salesman was repeatedly victimizing him resulting in serious problems, as his funds were limited. His son, as the nearest relative, worried how he would be able to negotiate giving assistance without threatening his father's sense of autonomy. His reluctance to intervene meant that the situation continued to deteriorate. Finally the daughter convinced her father to move closer to her family where she was

> able to gain his confidence, take care of his financial affairs, encourage more social activities and see that his nutritional needs were met. Although reluctant to leave his home of many years, it was his choice to make the move across the country and it was a success.

Lessons Learned

In order to preserve the right to make decisions about our own lives, we must project thoughts to the future. No matter how healthy we are at the present time, no matter how long we think we can manage our lives in the way we do now, there will come a time when we will probably not be able to on the same level. And, if experience is any indicator, many of us will not recognize that fact at the time. If we are prepared to accept less than favorable alternatives now before they are perceived as limits to our freedom and independence, we can feel that truly we have retained control of our lives.

Having been a part of this process several times, I am struck by how difficult it is for family members to know when to become involved in a parent or loved one's affairs. For the person being helped, the biggest obstacle to overcome appears to be fear. There are so many fears; fear of not enough money, of illness, most especially dementia, fear of the unexpected, of leaving the familiar, or, more importantly, of losing independence, of nursing homes or of becoming a problem to one's family and friends.

Many adult children with parents aging before their eyes go through several stages themselves before circumstances force problems to be addressed. First there is confidence that elderly parents are managing well without help. Then an accident or illness indicates increasing vulnerability. We are so reluctant to intervene and change the status quo that we are ourselves guilty of what is often called denial just as the person having the problems sometimes is. We worry even more if there are signs of confusion about financial affairs and frustration when we can't talk it over. Finally there is despair as we perceive increasingly poor health and clear signs of cognitive decline are affecting a loved one's well-being. Sometimes nothing can be done until the elderly person asks for help or someone else points out the necessity for intervention. Once the decision has been made to do so, using sensitivity to recognize and acknowledge a person's sense of self is important. For many of us who struggle to keep up with the demands of an already busy life, having our parents feel our gratitude and relief that they are willing to accept our help can be a daunting prospect.

Sometimes a Helping Hand is All that is Needed

When perceiving resistance in an attempt to help a parent or an elderly relative, we need to step back or move more slowly than we would like to in order to effect the changes *we* feel need to be made. As my siblings and I became more sensitive to and sympathetic with the emotions my mother was feeling, we were able to work together to come up with an acceptable solution but it was a long and frustrating process. Her reaction didn't look like fear, nor was it identified as such by my mother who we were trying to help but hindsight made me realize how perhaps we could have been more sensitive to such a possibility thus leading to a better way to present a solution.

Problem solving for someone else makes us think of the implications of our intervention. Being aware of such complex emotions will help us find a balance between effecting what we feel is a necessary change and respecting the autonomy of the person we're trying to assist. Someday if we should be in need, perhaps we will understand that being gracious in the acceptance of assistance when it is offered is an indication of our own confidence and control not necessarily the yielding of independence. Reminding ourselves of that fact is important as we move into the future.

> *In the last year of my mother's life, a plumbing incident in her house caused a gaping hole in the ceiling of the front hall. It was unsightly and perhaps even dangerous. Thinking I was helping her and with her reluctant acceptance, I lined up plasterers and*

painters to make the repairs. I offered to be there to oversee the work but when the workers arrived she refused to let them in the house. I was aggravated and frustrated and the work was not done until after she died. It took a long time for me to understand that she was asserting a need to be in charge of her own life as long as she could. She simply did not want the noise and disruption of such work being done in her house. Acknowledging that my actions were counter-productive, I had to reconcile the strength of her instinct to retain control with my own desire to solve the problem.

Resource

This is an organization that helps caregivers by providing information, a national information and referral service for local resources and best of all emotional support. They have a really impressive Website. I suggest consulting it for information for oneself whether as a caregiver or to help in covering all the issues of care giving before they are needed.

    Children of Aging Parents
    1609 Woodbourne RD, Suite 302A
    Levittown, PA 19057—800 227 7294

                      www.caps4caregivers.org

I have looked through many books for caregivers of the elderly and none of them covers more material better than this one. Easy to read format, a large range of solutions to the issues presented and good resources.

        HOW TO CARE for AGING PARENTS
    By Virginia Morris—Workman Publishing Company—1996—
ISBN 1-56305-435-3

A Checklist of Questions for Caregivers, Families and Ourselves

The following partial list of questions from the Website of the Children of Aging Parents is an important aid for lining up details to consider when caring for anyone, particularly an elderly relative. While reading, answer them for yourself especially if you are middle aged or older and keep asking them as you age or if you have a chronic illness or are living alone. There are some important issues to be addressed in planning for a time when we might need some help in the future.

General Issues

- Who will be the principal caregiver?
- What involvement will siblings have?
- Which responsibilities can be shared? By Whom? (Supervising medications, shopping, doctors, day care, etc.)
- Is there good communication between caregiver and elderly person?
- Do family members share feelings and information?

Financial and Legal

- What is the person's financial situation?
- Is there a list of assets, their value, and their locations?
- Is there a private pension? Is it mailed directly to a bank? Which one?
- What is the social security amount? Is it directly deposited? Where?
- Are there any other sources of income? Annuities, stocks, interest, IRA's, CD's, Safe deposit box?
- What are the debts? Mortgages, car payment?
- Is there a need to apply for SSI, Supplementary Security Income?
- Is medical coverage adequate?
- Is there a prescription plan? Long-term care insurance? Medicare? Medicaid?
- Has anyone consulted an eldercare attorney?
- Has the elderly person transferred any assets?

- What is the "time frame" in your state for transferring assets before being qualified for Medicaid?
- Is there a will, a living will, a power of attorney, and a durable power of attorney that lasts beyond incapacitation? Where are they kept?
- Is there an insurance policy? Where is it kept?

Housing

- What housing options are possible? Can the elderly person live alone?
- What about an assisted living facility?
- Is a nursing facility or a personal care facility needed?
- Is senior housing or shared housing an option?
- Is a life care community feasible?
- Has the person or family any "up-front money" available for some period of personal pay in a nursing home?

Physical Condition

- Has the person had a recent physical? Is there a family doctor? Has a geriatric assessment been ordered?
- What medications are being taken? By prescription? Over the counter?
- Ask the pharmacist or doctor if any medication interactions should be avoided. Ask if any meds should not be taken together. Any food avoided?

After Death

- Are there any pre-paid funeral expenses? Any specific funeral wishes?
- What funeral home? A viewing? A family plot?
- Cremation? Any specific desires?
- Can you discuss death with the person for whom you are

caring? Why not? Many of the elderly do not fear discussion of death.

Negotiating a Minefield—
Dealing with Ghosts of Relationships Past

Whether it is a partner with whom we have shared a marriage, a parent or dear friend who becomes needy, the ability to respond effectively will cause us to draw on strengths we never knew we had. The hardest part is to face changing the way things were before. Love, respect, devotion, trust, caring, benign neglect, generosity, suspicion, self-centeredness, independence, comfortable sense of self, anger and fear of dependence are all issues defining a relationship that even when it works well may be full of stress. Clearing up unresolved issues is a first step in finding peace and becoming a valuable resource for someone else.

Whatever the reason, the shifting of roles after decades of relative balance in any relationship can be emotionally unsettling and requires more patience than most people know how to provide. Without exception, the most difficult step to take is the one that crosses the line of someone else's personal independence.

The problem often does not lie in the giving of assistance or the care. The problem comes in the negotiation of what will be accepted and how to manage that within the framework of the potential caregiver's life.

Few of us envision a time when chronic confusion could hinder our ability to manage a checkbook, an accident cause incapacity, or lifestyle decisions taken when young or middle aged, affect our ability to take care of ourselves later in life. The problem is that such things do happen and making someone understand that he or she needs help can be difficult. Knowing when to intervene or how much help to give is often determined by instinct and by what will be accepted.

Since few of us are experienced in understanding all the problems, recognizing and finding solutions to what we encounter can be frustrating. In my own attempt to help my mother, each day brought another issue we were not sure how to solve. There were discussions and disagreements and misunderstandings but we did come up with an appropriate system for her.

When Some Nursing Care is Necessary

Before discharge from most hospitals, the social services or discharge planner's office will have been notified by the doctor about the level of nursing needed by the patient. On meeting with the patient they will, in most cases, provide lists of qualified agencies or facilities if a family member cannot provide the nursing care required. This is only a place to start and is by no means a guarantee that other, more suitable services are not available.

In our experience, the recommendations made by the hospital have been good in two instances and unsuccessful in one. When the system works well, one can get a lot of support for finding a way through the complicated mix of requirements and advice, particularly if dealing with Medicare. It helps in the search to know what we are looking for, what we can afford and what is covered by an insurance or medical plan. Some hospitals do an excellent job of preparing the patient for release and the after-care required. For all of its detractors, Medicare services for post release from a hospital are in most cases helpful and surprisingly effective. As the relatives who were helping a patient, we were grateful when the system worked. It led us through the care requirements and showed us what we had to do to meet them. I have complained, like many others I know, about the bureaucracy and the paperwork but I give them high marks for the assistance we did receive.

What to do When Things Don't Work as Well as They Should

Anecdotal experiences recounted by friends who have been

through it clearly express the frustration of dealing with a system that refuses appropriate care for patients too ill to fight the battle for themselves. Admission to a rehabilitation or acute care facility for recovery from surgery, stroke, and other serious medical events is sometimes difficult to qualify for. It may be obvious to anyone providing care to the patient that skilled nursing is required in the name of safety and recovery but that does not always mean it will be provided. When that level of support and care is not available at home, then another way must be found to get the services needed.

- There is usually some warning before a patient must be discharged because Medicare or one's insurance will not pay for additional time. Sometimes if a case can be made that there is nowhere else for the patient to go on short notice, the system will relent for a short time. When we felt that discharge was premature, we got all the facts of our relative's condition so they could be documented and successfully resubmitted the request.
- When all else fails, we have to learn how to fight for what we believe is right. Appeal the process at every level from the doctor to the social worker assigned, to the insurance carrier, the HMO or Medicare person we talk with on the phone, the supervisor and back again. Persistence with verifiable facts can sometimes win the day

---

RESOURCE

The National Council on Aging has a Website with a questionnaire to help the elderly or caregivers find out if they qualify for benefits, which range from home health care to discounts on prescriptions.

www.benefitscheckup.org

Check the local phone directory for the National Council on Aging for more information if you do not have Internet.

Levels of Care Available

Once the decision has been made to discharge a patient from the hospital the search begins for a facility most able to supply appropriate care for the patient's needs. There are several alternatives that could be suggested.

A Transitional, Acute Care or Rehabilitation Facility

Care in this type of facility is designed to assist the patient after a hospital stay where care focuses on diagnosis and treatment of acute problems such as stroke, fractures or hip and knee replacements. Short-term admission with skilled nursing care, rehabilitation, physical, and occupational therapy services is provided where one can relearn the skills necessary to live independently again.

Things to Look For

- Pay attention to word of mouth. We can usually tell a lot about a place from what former patients, their families and even employees say about it. I have observed that management and ownership change frequently with resultant swings in services provided so it is important to get timely information on any place being considered.
- In looking into a local rehabilitation center for a friend recovering from a stroke, we found the corporation running it had several other facilities in the area. The one we were investigating had an excellent reputation, which proved to be accurate, but another owned by the same corporation only 10 miles away proved to be sub-standard. While she was there, the management changed hands with resultant confusion and lapses in care.
- Are medical and professional staffs up to industry standards? Some doctors helped us to get that information for our

patient, but our best information came from a geriatric case manager who gave us her professional evaluation of the facilities we were referred to.

In some cases, Medicare will pay for residence and treatment in such a facility as long as there is a possibility of improvement in function and health. (True at this writing) This should be an incentive to the patient to be serious about prescribed physical and occupational therapy requirements because rules governing the prolonging of residence are strict. **Note:** Depression, which sometimes follows surgery or serious illness, could influence personal efforts and ability to get the most from rehabilitation therapy so be sure the patient gets attention for such a condition should it be needed.

- Most facilities are operating on a tight budget, both profit and nonprofit, therefore staff and services are usually at a bare minimum sufficient only to ensure safety and hopefully positive results for the recovering patient. Do not expect special attention.
- Find out if admission will be on a floor with people who suffer from some form of dementia. Patients with this problem require different attention and security procedures so one may find freedom limited unnecessarily.
- Hire an off-duty caregiver approved by the facility to give a few hours of specialized attention several days a week or daily if possible. Staff in rehabilitation or nursing facilities is able to give only the minimum care required by the condition of the patient. What a difference it can make to one's comfort and well being to have someone take extra effort helping a patient to eat, give a bath or even a back rub!

Types of Private Home Health/Nursing Care

The doctor may decide that care in the home is preferable to that which would be received in a rehabilitation or nursing facility. If that is the case there are several alternatives available

- *A Companion/Sitter* does general housecleaning, cooking and in-home supervision. He/she can give some medications and can assist the patient with personal care. This person often has no formal training but usually has experience in caring for people who need it at home. They can be hired by the hour although there may be a required minimum of four or more hours.
- *A Certified nursing assistant, CNA* has had some training in a professional facility, (often a nursing home) and should have a state certificate. A CNA can provide personal care and is taught to assist patients with normal functions. They may touch, move, bathe and administer most medications by agreement with the doctor and the family.
- *A Licensed practical nurse (LPN)* generally has a two-year degree from a college, has received specialized training and has a state license. LPN's are qualified to touch, move and assist patients who require specialized care as well as administer medication.
- *Registered nurses (RN)* have from two to four years or more of training, are licensed by the state, and have specialized training. An RN can provide skilled nursing care as well as all the services listed above.
- *An Intravenous therapy nurse* is an RN who provides highly specialized and technical care dealing with intravenous therapy. (This is the giving of medications through the blood system or other internal, artificial method.)
- *Visiting nurse* providers supplement other home care arrangements where oversight and some limited nursing is required. A visiting nurse is an RN who works in cooperation with the doctor to provide necessary care and in some cases supervises general home care arrangements.
- *Hospice care* in the home is a unique program providing

nursing for the terminally ill patient and support services for both patient and family. Special training is required for caregivers, and may include CNA's, visiting nurses, doctors, chaplains and counselors who help the patient and family through the grieving process.
- *Respite care* is temporary care provided by a person with the required level of training relieving the usual caregiver for hours, days or weeks.
- *Supervised adult day care* offers services such as health assessment, social activities and therapy on a daily basis in an "away from home" setting for the Alzheimer's or dementia patient.
- *A Home Health Care Manager or Geriatric Care Manager* can provide the services needed for evaluating the level of care needed, the hiring of caregivers and the management of schedules and general oversight of the patient's needs.

Finding the Best Caregiver

Once an assessment has been made of the level of care needed, the first step is to involve the person requiring the care in each facet of the process, if this is possible. The next step is to find the best and most efficient provider of the required care at a cost that is acceptable. Some insurance plans will require that home health care workers be supplied by an approved agency. This in no way guarantees better service or more highly trained personnel.

- Be clear on what is expected of any home care agency and then be prepared to press a case for that level of care with the agency, the insurance company and any regulatory organization.
- Understand that hiring an agency to provide personnel is only the first step in an ongoing process of evaluation and supervision in order to receive the best care.
- Network with friends and friends of friends who have had

to solve the same problem. Ask for referrals and always follow up on references.

Skill in the caring business is important but skill without a cheerful and positive nature is useless.

When arranging care for my mother on an "around the clock" basis in her own home, we found it was a good idea to check on caregivers at different hours of the day and night until we were sure that the fit was a good one. We worked through a recommended agency thinking that paying a higher fee ensured better service and well-trained workers but found to our distress that this was not always the case. Many of the caregivers worked second jobs so if the relief caregiver didn't show up on time for the next shift, there was often no one to fill in on short notice even though the agency was supposed to provide a replacement in a timely fashion. Not all caregivers were kind and caring. At one time we found by accident that my mother was being emotionally abused. She had not complained because she was afraid she would be moved to a nursing home if she did.

Caregivers who work in home health care through an agency often receive low salaries, no health or vacation benefits and little job security. The wonder is that there are any well-trained, compassionate and intelligent caregivers but there are many. It sometimes takes trial and error to find the best person for both patient and caregiver, but when it works, the peace and happiness it brings are worth everything. For us, a solution was to hire one worker who suited my mother's needs the best as an independent contractor and she found the others to fill out the schedule. We paid a little more than the agency had paid each of the caregivers but they, in turn, received more take home pay because the fee went entirely to them. The biggest benefit was that our mother received loyalty and reliable service in return.

Resource

This has been recommended as a good book for both the caregiver and recipient of long-term care.

    Taking Charge—Overcoming the Challenges of Long-Term Illness
        By Irene Pollin and Susan K. Golant—Times Books, New York—
                ISBN 0-812-92258-1

The Competent Caregiver: A Guide to Hiring Care in the Home Independently
        By Elizabeth Ducasse—1st Books Library—ISBN 1-588-20292-5

Putting a System of Full or Part Time Home Health Care to Work

In setting up full time live-in care for a relative recently, we used the advice of a geriatric case manager who provided applicants for the job and who gave us invaluable advice about the hiring process and practical things we had to know to make the system work smoothly. If the patient has long term care insurance, see what the terms are. Some policies allow a family member to be paid for providing care. This is also something to keep in mind when purchasing a Long Term Care Insurance policy.

Decide which type of system will work best for patient and family

- Care by supportive friends, relatives and/or spouse
- Workers who are supervised and paid by an agency or by the patient.
- Independent contractors, who work for the patient, are paid for and supervised by the same.
- Informal support system supported by volunteers.
- Someone has to take responsibility for supervising that care is consistent. One person should be the contact with the doctor and with the family member.

Managing a Home Health Care System

We have had experience with using an agency for home care, hiring workers supplied by an agency, and independent contracting with caregivers. Finding the right mix for caregiver and patient is a time consuming and sometimes discouraging project. It is rarely as simple as picking up the phone and having someone show up. Hiring caregivers, dealing with the payroll, insurance and supervision issues is a full time job. In most cases, a patient cannot be expected to concentrate on recovery and running a home health care system at the same time.

This type of system is often more affordable than dealing with an agency. Continuity and the ability to count on someone are important to a patient who is being cared for and also to the one responsible for the schedule. On the negative side, a pleasant personality and even positive references are not a guarantee of good patient care so an experienced person might have several false starts before finding the right match. It is difficult for an individual to find out about a caregiver's reputation for reliability and honesty. More importantly, it takes an experienced person to know how to do a check for criminal activity or abuse. Very time consuming.

- Understand the difference between custodial, semi-skilled and critical care nursing.
- Follow up on references when interviewing applicants. Nothing is a guarantee of perfect service but they can give an indication of trouble areas. Ask if the person is bonded and find out what experience the candidate has in caring for the patient's particular type of need.
- Find an agency that will provide people who are bonded, have been checked for a criminal background, and with whom the agency has had experience. Such assistance will be helpful in supplying back-up personnel when needed. Some will give advice in setting up a financial and oversight system for one's own management.

- Pay adequately with promise of increases at regular intervals. Care giving is a skill and the happiness of a loved one is so dependent on the quality of care received that it is false economy to think of saving money by pinching pennies in this area. Remember special incentives for holiday care as most of the workers have families also.
- Spell out exactly what the caregiver's responsibilities are so there can be no misplaced expectations. Find out from others or an agency what the usual requirements of such care giving are then adapt them to the situation.
- Remove valuables such as jewelry, silver, and firearms in the interest of the patient AND the caregiver. Inventory what is left or make a videotape record of each room in the house before any one is hired. Inform the caregiver of this and ask them to list any gifts given them by the patient. Be aware that patients with dementia sometimes hide valuables, can't find them or give them away and then accuse the caregiver of stealing. Have the telephone company place a block on the telephone for anything but basic local service.
- Establish a policy on caregiver visitors and strict guidelines on alcohol use and smoking especially when they are living in the house. A caregiver's friend was found to be stealing items from our relative's house. Although the caregiver may not have known about it, the visitor should not have been there.
- See that the caregiver has all the tools he or she needs to effectively care for the patient. This means safety proofing the house, (an evaluation can be done by a social worker) emergency lighting in the case of power failures, phone numbers of people to reach for emergencies, etc.
- Periodically inquire of both patient and caregiver if there are any changes that could be made to ensure better care or smoother running of the household. Just asking the question sometimes eliminates an irritant before it becomes a problem.
- When managing care for a terminally ill patient, make sure everyone in the household understands the policy on medical

- Keep careful track of expenses by requiring receipts for every purchase and where there are monthly accounts with a store or pharmacy check charges frequently. It is not a good idea for the patient to be the person paying the bills as there is too much possibility for fraud, possible pressure from the caregiver to buy too much and difficulty in providing oversight. There are trustworthy agencies that can be contracted with to pay the bills, do the payroll and keep track of expenses to be sure there are no excesses.
- Check that homeowner's insurance covers people employed in the home.
- Set up a daily logbook that has the following;

    1. Responsibilities of caregiver and supervisor
    2. Emergency numbers, relatives and friends of the patient, their numbers, pharmacies and doctors
    3. Person covering shifts, dates and times
    4. Condition of patient, medications given and times, activities, etc.
    5. Visitors and gifts brought
    6. Section for listing of repairs, supplies needed or things to be brought to the supervisor's attention
    7. A pocket for keeping receipts of all purchases and expenses
    8. A reminder placed on the inside of the front cover of the logbook that all items in the house have been inventoried and a video record made of the contents. It is for protection and benefit of the caretaker and patient therefore gifts given to the caregiver should be noted in the logbook. (This does not mean that things won't disappear because they often do. In many cases the

patient either gives them away or actually hides them for safekeeping then can't remember where they are.)

Note: When caregivers are required to keep records, the person supervising should read them frequently to encourage careful note keeping and because it is a good way to spot previously undetected changes in the patient's condition.

Searching for a Full Service Agency

The biggest surprise for me in arranging care for my mother when she returned from the hospital and needed full time nursing was that signing up with an agency that supplied home health care services did not mean that all our problems were solved. Supervision and oversight on a continual basis was required to assure good care giving. In some cases the persons assigned were not adequately trained or even reliable. Having a Hospice approved agency was also no guarantee that a caregiver would be the best match.

- Search for an agency that has received high marks from friends or social workers of local hospitals. State or city Department of the Aging offices should have records of any complaints and lists of home health care agencies.
- Have a clear understanding of the contract made with an agency or the caregiver. Understand what duties are the caregiver's and what will have to be taken care of by someone else.
- Do not delay reporting concerns about problems with the level of care, personality conflicts or suspicion of possible emotional or physical abuse, theft or fraud to the agency.
- Know what it takes to provide the best care.
- Visits from relatives and friends should occur at unexpected times to ensure that appropriate care is being provided all the time. Frequent supervision and oversight are necessary.

- The worker should know how to reach a family member overseeing the care at all times.
- Remember that caregivers are human. As explained above, they work under trying conditions, have little job security, often no health insurance and although they provide a vital service are not paid very well. Even with all of those problems, most of them with whom I have had contact are intelligent, caring and skilled people. Care giving at any level is a job requiring specialized skills. One must have inordinate patience, personal initiative, the ability to respond to emergencies, the flexibility to get along with different personalities including some which, even under the best of circumstances are not particularly likeable, and an inexhaustible supply of good will. There may be some who will disappoint but the vast majority deserve respect and understanding even when personal needs intrude on a smooth running system.
- Never forget the patient. Personality conflicts if not resolved can have a serious effect on care and recovery. When someone is confined to a bed, a house, a severely limited life, focus is naturally on the care received and those providing it therefore personality becomes a big issue. Always listen to a patient's complaints about inadequate care, even those who have some cognitive impairment because there may be some truth to it.
- Establish a clear chain of command especially where there are many family members in the area.
- Plan frequent unannounced visits.
- Keep eyes and ears open. When we were involved with the care of a relative, we came to trust our noses, our eyes and our instincts when checking details like cleanliness of both patient and caregiver.
- Find time to talk to both caregiver and patient privately to find out how things are going. It is my experience that many patients, particularly the elderly, will not express complaints or concerns as they fear being placed in a nursing home or

because they don't want to trouble anyone. Sometimes an objective observer is better at evaluating how things are going.

The positive reasons for having a full service agency are that background checks, bonding of employees, and reliability of skill levels should be guaranteed. An attempt to make a good match with the patient from a pool of applicants, taking care of payroll and paperwork and timely replacement of caretakers when necessary, are only some of the features usually provided. The downside is that care supplied by an agency can be expensive. This means the agency keeps a large part of the fee and the worker, depending on experience, sometimes receives no more than minimum wage. Workers often do not get health benefits, vacation pay or pension therefore job loyalty is not always high. Consistent level of performance is hard to find, substitute workers may not always be provided when personal emergencies occur to scheduled caregivers and they often do.

Keep Avenues of Communication Open with All the Family

Usually there is one person who assumes responsibility for overseeing the care of an elderly relative, either by default, because of proximity or through personal choice. It is important that the rest of the family be kept up to date with what is happening and that they be given opportunities to assist in the home care. Keeping everyone up-to-date helps to establish a continuity of concerned care if something should happen to the primary caregiver.

One way to keep everyone informed and involved in the process is to issue a report and up-date it on a regular basis. We kept a file with pertinent details of what was known about medical, financial and personal needs in an obvious place so that someone could step in if we were on vacation or became ill ourselves.

Information to Share with Relatives

- A brief summary of the person's condition and situation

- Things that can be done to bring cheer or comfort
- Reminder of up-coming birthdays, anniversaries, etc.
- Where help could be used.
- An update on the giving away, temporary storage or sale of items from the house or estate if it is pertinent

Suppose I am the Patient and My Partner is the Caregiver?

Managing one's own illness is difficult enough. Struggling to retain control of our lives and doing everything we can to keep from being a worry to those closest to us can uncover emotional issues that need to be resolved, not only for us but for the persons caring for us. It is our responsibility to know ourselves well enough to realize when help is needed and to be willing to seek it. If we are overcome with emotions and/or depression, we must have the courage to seek professional help. A spiritual advisor, wise friend, a doctor, or a therapist can be of help in addressing issues that divert energy from the effort to get well. Support for the caregiver starts with proper training and continues with an understanding of what is being asked of the caregiver. Statistics and anecdotal information show that men have more difficulty learning to become caregivers, especially when having to deal with actual nursing activities such as bathing someone else, and assisting with personal care while at the same time managing to cook meals and keeping the house running. But I have seen loving and expert caregivers who were men so I know they can do it. If we can afford it, hiring extra help now and then to spell the caregiver would ease the load. But most important, understand the pressures of being a caregiver and don't expect perfection.

Resource

To read: This is a beautifully written description of a journey into the world of dependency . . . from both sides.

Counting on Kindness
  By Wendy Lustbader—Free Press—ISBN 0029195160

This is a not-for-profit association of spousal caregivers. It offers support for the wives, husbands, and partners of chronically ill or disabled people. They have lists of support groups nationwide and sponsors recreational respite opportunities.
  The Well Spouse Foundation
  63 W. Main St., Suite H
  Freehold, NJ 07728—800 838-0879
      www.wellspouse.org—info@wellspouse.org

For many of us, a loved one's health problems are harder to cope with emotionally than if they were our own. For that reason, it is important to consider that keeping the person giving the care healthy is as important as recovery and care for the loved one. The formula for effective care giving is different for each of us but the personal investment brought to the equation is what makes it all come together.

Confidence that care will be consistently good and that the patient does not have to adjust to unfamiliar faces or have people coming and going in his or her own house are two of the biggest benefits of such a system. The downside is that there is no getting away from the responsibility, the emotional and physical drain of both patient and caregiver that comes from changing roles brought on by increasing dependency and the daily necessities of caring for a loved one. If the caregiver has a full time job, giving up that income may put family finances in jeopardy. Something to remember is that the Family and Medical Leave Act allows workers at companies employing 50 or more people to take up to 12 weeks of unpaid leave each year to care for a child, spouse or parent with a serious illness and to return to their former job or an equivalent one.

- Don't let anxiety be immobilizing. Create order if there is

chaos. Assign a priority to the problems being faced and deal with them in turn. Concentrate on doing what is necessary to get through each day.
- Learn how to accept help when it is offered. Select those tasks that would make the day better but do not require specialized knowledge or training.
- Consider hiring a caretaker on a part-time basis for a few days a month if it can be afforded or ask a friend to step in and help now and then. The cost of threatening our own emotional and physical health is too high when it comes to long-term care-giving.
- Fight the isolation that comes from dealing with a serious illness. Social contact and interaction are essential for everyone. Contact a church or community group to help with respite care when needed now and then.
- Make visits by friends interesting and fun for all concerned. Think about what it is that will help the conversation along with things of mutual interest. Making the effort to be a host is often difficult for someone who is not feeling well. At the same time it is more comfortable for the person visiting if there are thing to do such as opening the mail together or reading from a particularly loved book, talking politics or reading the daily newspaper together. Quiet companionship is equally as comforting as active stimulation and can be more restful for the patient.
- Develop a plan for emergency and long-term care if the primary caregiver should become ill or incapacitated.

Resource

Although I have not read this myself, it comes highly recommended.
The Comfort of Home: An Illustrated Step-by-Step Guide for Caregivers,
Second Edition
By Marcia M. Meyer—Care Trust Publications LLC—ISBN 0-9664767-0-0

Caring for Someone From a Long Way Away

I often receive phone calls from friends who are in the position of finding care for a parent or relative who lives a state or even a continent away. I have seen them respond to a crisis by dropping everything, taking leave from a job, making arrangements for their own children to be cared for and traveling to deal with a situation for which they are unprepared. When living far away from those we love, the signs of increasing need may be difficult to discern. Sometimes there are a few clues like confusion on the telephone or suggestions from the person's neighbors that things are not going well. Denial plays a role in our unwillingness to believe that the need really exists just as it does in acceptance by the person who is failing that independence may be threatened.

In most cases a relative arrives on the scene, perhaps far from home, assesses the problem and seeks out a series of solutions that appear to make the most sense. The person needing the help sometimes doesn't want to accept any of them, much less agrees that there is any reason to. Neighbors and friends are consulted and press for solutions, sometimes because they do not wish to take responsibility for what they see as a deteriorating situation. The difficulty is that, in the rush and single-minded wish to solve the problem, there is often little time to listen to hidden meanings, to make sense of what is being seen and what friends have been saying. This is the moment when we wish we had been talking to this loved one long before now about prospects for the future. If I can put myself in the position of that parent, I may find it is easier to understand how what appears to be a perfectly satisfactory solution to me could cause a negative response and stubborn resistance.

A Geriatric Care Manager can Help

When faced with this type of problem as a concerned relative or friend, I suggest that, rather than forcing a solution, a better strategy is to remove oneself from the equation and get a third party to evaluate what needs to be done and to suggest alternatives. This is not an inexpensive process and there is no guarantee that it will be successful in resolving the problem but it is a place to start. A care manager is an advocate for the patient and might be a social worker, registered nurse, psychologist or Certified Nursing Assistant trained in the needs of the elderly. He or she should be well acquainted with the services available in the community and can even do the interviewing, hiring and supervision of caregivers for home health care if it is necessary. Professional assistance in the selection of a nursing facility is invaluable particularly if the need is far away from other family members. A care manager can also provide regular oversight to be sure that care is appropriate and the patient's rights are observed. Other services that can be provided are bill paying, crisis intervention, escort services to the doctor and oversight in a hospital or nursing home to be sure that care is adequate. Care is tailored to the individual and communication with the family keeps everyone informed. In cases of financial need some people qualify for assistance by community services and can be assessed at little or no cost. There is usually a long waiting list and the qualifying criteria are strict but it is well worth trying.

- Seek a qualified person or agency through the national organization for such managers, the local Area Agency on Aging, or the Eldercare Locator.
- How much experience has this person had with geriatric cases?
- Ask for a clear definition of the services being provided and ask for a written copy.
- Ask if the care manager is licensed or credentialed in a particular specialty such as social workers, RN, counselor, etc. Ask for references and then follow up on them.
- Ask the person to be specific about costs and fees to be charged.
- Will the geriatric care manager present the evaluation and options to the person needing help? Even those suffering

from the first signs of dementia syndrome may be more willing to accept the conclusion that they must have help when it is given by an independent professional rather than a family member.
- Set up a system of concerned oversight by asking friends who live nearby to visit often and then check with them frequently for their opinion of the condition of the patient and the care being given.

RESOURCE

Just to remind, this organization can locate help anywhere in the country through their referral system.

ELDERCARE LOCATOR—800 677-1116—*www.eldercare.gov/*
Hours of operation : Monday—Friday 9AM—8 PM Eastern Time

If looking for a geriatric care manager go to the Web site of the National Association of Professional Geriatric Care Managers for everything you need to know about selection. They also have a list of members from which to choose.

www.caremanager.org

Searching for a Nursing Home is a Complicated Process

There are few individuals my age or older who do not have a horror of being forced into a nursing home someday. We have seen that dread and fear in our own parents and heard them say again and again, "Please let me go in my sleep." From my interviews I find that it's not a fear of death in such a place that often disquiets a person, it is fear of dying alone. It is the possibility of a prolonged existence wrapped in the cocoon of an unfamiliar environment, isolation from family and friends and dependency on strangers for the most elementary tasks of daily living that preys on one's mind.

It doesn't have to be this way

Each of us can make ourselves knowledgeable about the options available and then see that our family knows what we have learned and decided before it becomes necessary. What few of us wish to think about is that someday, even when relatively young, we could become incapacitated to such an extent that we could not make our wishes known. It is at this point that our friends and relatives would be relieved of the responsibility of guessing what we wanted if we had faced the possibility of such an eventuality ahead of time.

I have been in some of the most highly rated church-run, corporate and/or privately administered modern nursing homes and been appalled by the conditions. On the other hand, I have seen care given in a cheerful, clean environment that had an air of what might be called decayed gentility where all patients were treated with affection and respect. Whether a facility is profit or nonprofit is not necessarily an indicator of the care to be found in such places but personal observation, word of mouth and information from staff who work there is always more valuable than an advertising brochure.

For those of us looking for such a facility for someone else, the search for an appropriate place and the attempt to see that care is consistently good once admitted, requires perseverance and takes a lot of work.

- Know something about the organization being researched. Is it nonprofit, a corporation, a hospital, a religious organization or privately owned?
- Check with local or state agencies for information on nursing homes to see if there are complaints listed or outstanding deficiencies noted.
- Go to visit. Ask questions

    1. Ask to see facilities on the floor where admission would be.
    2. Are the rooms cheerful and large enough? Are there

any private rooms? Is there a bath for each room? Are there provisions for privacy?
3. Does the facility smell and look clean?
4. When walking around the halls, do staff members know the residents by name and do they address them with respect?
5. Is there a barber or hairdresser available?
6. When the weather is moderate, is there a place for residents to sit outside?
7. Is visiting allowed at any hour? If so, check in the off hours and see if residents are well cared for at those times.

The Staff is Key to Comfort and a Sense of Well Being

- Do they look cheerful and do they treat the patients with real interest and affection?
- What is the ratio of patients per caregiver? Per therapist?
- How many of the caregivers are hired on an hourly basis, how many supplied by an agency, and what is the turnover rate for this level of staff?
- Do all employees have benefits such as sick pay, vacation time or health insurance? Try to find a staff member who will answer questions and ask him or her what is most difficult about the job and whether there is a feeling of being appreciated by the institution. An unhappy or underpaid staff member directly relates to the level of care one can expect to find.

Resource

We have used this service to evaluate nursing homes for a relative and found it to be informative. The figures do not tell the whole story and cannot be a substitute of an on-site visit.

www.medicare.gov

We Should Never Accept Abuse for Ourselves or for Anyone Else

Abuse of a vulnerable patient is the dark side of the caregiver picture. Opportunities for mistreatment exist not only in a hospital or nursing home, but also in a private home with a hired health care worker or even a family member who may be over stressed, resentful of the responsibility or not suitable as a caregiver. For those who have been living the caregiver experience day in and day out, particularly with a patient who suffers from dementia or Alzheimer's disease, the line between feeling overwhelmed and slipping into out-of-control frustration is very thin.

A person who is housebound or bedridden with a serious or chronic illness is particularly vulnerable in these situations even if not confused or verbally incommunicative. Discovering and documenting abuse of any kind is very difficult and often plausible explanations can be given for what appears to be physical evidence

Know What Constitutes Abuse

- *Physical* Examples range from striking with the hands or an object, withholding food, dentures or glasses to pinching, hair pulling, and rough handling during bathing, toileting or other procedures. Burning, physically restraining, pushing, shoving are extreme abuse. Over medication in order to make someone more tractable is also a form of abuse. Be aware that clothing or bedclothes may hide signs of abuse.
- *Emotional* Withholding pleasant activities, personal verbal attacks lowering self-esteem, threats of physical harm, treating an adult as if he or she were a misbehaving child, or isolating someone from friends and family are some of the ways patients can be abused.
- *Theft and Fraud* Valuables, small personal items may disappear from the home or room. A patient who controls the checkbook can be misled into signing checks for

unspecified amounts or excessive charges are made for unneeded services. Unauthorized use of the telephone is considered theft of services.

A patient or the person responsible for someone who is being cared for must be a careful consumer of caregiver services. Everyone has the right to expect at the minimum, adequate, appropriate care from the staff being paid to provide the service. Understand that abuse, although not a frequent problem *can* happen.

- Caregivers are human but also very busy, particularly in a nursing home. A visitor, family member or friend who is concerned about a patient can find out what the procedure is for registering complaints and then be a part of the solution. Visiting often and at unexpected times helps to create an atmosphere of caring and helps the staff in its care of the patient. In many cases it makes their efforts easier by raising spirits of all concerned.
- Know what constitutes the minimum requirements for care of a patient by the institution or agency with which they are involved. In a home health care situation, establish on the first day what duties are expected of the caregiver. It is helpful to post the list of duties in the room used by the caregivers or in the logbook kept daily of the patient's care if it is in the home.
- Proving that a problem exists can be very difficult and takes listening skills. Caregivers or attendants in many nursing homes and hospitals are usually given responsibility for a lot of patients. The patient may be making unfair demands and not understand the level of care able to be provided in such a setting. Providers often feel they are unappreciated by the nursing home and the patients. Being aware of the stress under which they operate can help motivate one to be sympathetic and perhaps realistic about what level of care is adequate.

- Listen to the patient. Some patients with dementia syndrome or Alzheimer's disease may complain of ill treatment when there is no proof of such being the case. Do not assume that it is all a figment of imagination. Come to visit at unexpected times, check to see the reaction of the patient to different caregivers, and see whether he or she is well groomed and clean whenever visiting.
- Talk with the caregivers.

    1. Do they express an interest in the patient?
    2. Does the agency, nursing home or hospital staff respond to concerns and have time to answer questions about the patient's care?

- It never hurts to bring the staff a treat now and then. A batch of cookies, or fresh fruit given to the nursing staff in the patient's name is unexpected and can be a great morale booster.
- Are visits encouraged at any time? If so, is the patient's room clean and is it odor free? Ask family members of other patients how they feel about the care.
- Keep in mind that incontinent patients require frequent attention and busy staff may not be able to attend to their needs immediately but should move to take care of the problem when notified. It is when the inattention occurs over a long period or more than occasionally that notice has to be taken before health issues emerge.

One way we solved the problem of avoiding abuse for an elderly relative was to have her long-time housekeeper stay on as a geriatric care manager. She came at unexpected times of the day or night to check on her friend and on the pretext of helping the attendant, would have an opportunity to check her body for bedsores, signs of abuse or other physical problems. She would sit for a visit and listen to complaints to see if she needed to do more frequent or closer observation. Although she was not trained to be a geriatric care manager, she had the decided advantage of knowing and being respected by the patient and had a proven record of loving concern for the patient.

Hospice is Another Word for End of Life Caring

Most of us have heard of Hospice. It is identified as a type of care, which gives comfort and support to patients and their families when a serious illness is no longer responding to treatments designed to cure it thus considered terminal. In order to fully understand Hospice, you have to have seen it in action or experienced it. The ability to ease pain with compassion and provide dignity to the dying patient at the same time as counseling family members and friends is truly unique. It is a team oriented concept where doctors, nurses, home health care workers, volunteers and family members come together to attend to the medical, emotional, social and spiritual needs of a dying patient. The Hospice team knows far more about the necessity for adequate pain relief than the usual primary doctor and it is their mandate to make the patient pain-free, alert and peaceful. Being assigned to Hospice care is not a death sentence. It is an acknowledgement that end of life passage can be a time of fulfillment, of peace, and of reconciliation. No one needs to die alone or in pain. In some cases, there is a process called *terminal sedation* that is perfectly legal but not often talked about by hospitals or doctors where a terminal patient in terrible pain can be kept in a sleep-like state and given high doses of pain medication. He or she can be awakened as needed but is otherwise peaceful. It is something to discuss with one's doctor if suffering from a terminal illness.

80% of Hospice care is provided in the home or in Hospice nursing homes. Respite care and in-patient facilities are offered in some locations.

Resource

This book gives such a clear and sympathetic vision of life affirming spirit and a description of Hospice services.

Signs of Life—A memoir of Dying and Discovery
By Tim Brookes—Times Books/Random House 1997—
ISBN 0-8129-2468-1

I found the best description of Hospice on the Internet. This website has a very useful and extensive list of resources for organizations that could be helpful in providing services to people who need them.

www.hospicefoundation.org

Look in a telephone directory for the local number of Hospice in your area to get more information.

CHAPTER SIX

UNDERSTANDING DEPRESSION AND MEMORY LOSS

Staying healthy emotionally requires knowledge of one-self, the sensitivity to recognize when help is needed and the skill to know how to find it. It means that we become as familiar with symptoms and treatment of emotional disorders as we would any other illness and that we cultivate the wisdom to help someone else find a way through depression or a safe path through dementia.

With advances in detection and treatment, depression, which so crippled the generations before us, is now being given the attention it deserves. Because I have been intimately involved with friends of several age groups who have had clinical depression, I have learned that early awareness and diagnosis makes successful treatment a much more likely prospect than in years past. I have found that there are many factors that can cause memory loss and depression and that each one can cause the other. I have learned from experts in the field of geriatric psychology and psychiatry that Alzheimer's Disease is treatable although not curable at the moment, and that advances in the field offer many promising avenues for postponing the most debilitating effects of AD, strategies for living independently longer and even someday, a cure. I have learned that a diagnosis of dementia is not necessarily the end of hope and that, if diagnosed early, the learning of "coping skills" can help someone manage daily chores even though there are increasing deficits in cognitive ability. In December of 2001, Medicare acknowledged the efficacy of treatment for AD patients by electing to reimburse patients suffering from AD who have been given physical and mental therapy treatments, which have been shown to help slow the effects of the illness.

Depression is No Longer a "Hidden" Illness

Many people feel that aging and growing sad are inevitable partners. The fact is that depression is not a normal state for anyone and is considered one of the most treatable conditions doctors encounter. Symptoms of depression can come on so slowly that they seem always to have been there. Unfortunately, in dealing with severe depression, it's a little like falling down a well... You may not know what is happening or how you got there but the chances are you can't get yourself out again without some help.

A Word of Caution about Diagnosis

Sometimes a primary care physician will fail to recognize depression in a patient who has it. Clinical depression is a serious disabling illness that affects mood, thought, physical health and behavior. Often symptoms are unrecognized for many years by both the person suffering from depression and close associates or family members. Complicating a diagnosis is that many doctors are not trained to recognize the signs of depression, particularly in the aging.

In discussing their problems with the doctor, some people will identify physical symptoms rather than mentioning emotional issues not understanding the interrelationship of the two. Many will make an effort to "rise to the occasion" during visits to the doctor therefore it is important that a physician be experienced in recognizing the signs and symptoms of depression. Even when depression has become acute, some doctors are not familiar with it or may be as puzzled as the patient about what is wrong. If the condition is identified, it is sometimes not adequately treated as the doctor may opt to relieve the symptoms but not the underlying causes.

> *I saw first hand how this could happen when accompanying an older friend to the doctor who suffered many of the symptoms listed below. The physician patted him reassuringly on the back and said that there was nothing wrong with him but that he ought to expect to feel tired or down now and then since he was well into his 80s. His prescription was to buck up his spirits and move on. The perception that the pain he felt was what everyone his age should have to live with was reinforced and therefore getting him in to see a specialist wasn't possible until the symptoms became so severe that he was unable to take care of himself.*
>
> *I suspect my mother suffered for many years with depression but because of an iron will, and the ability to deny she had any problem and to mislead her doctor, she was never treated for it. She was put through a number of unpleasant and expensive tests searching for a physical cause for her discomfort only to end up frustrated because no explanation for her symptoms was found. Luckily, she did not become incapacitated by depression but she carried a heavy load when she could have found relief with the proper treatment.*

Research confirms that poor mental health significantly affects physical health and recovery rates from serious illness. It is estimated that nearly two thirds of those who experience depression do not get the help they need although treatment could alleviate the symptoms of more than 80% of them. The stigma that surrounds depression, particularly in the minds of people who lived through the Great Depression and the World Wars, keeps many of them from seeking treatment. It was widely believed that depression was a moral and physical failing and that if one were strong enough, it could be overcome by personal will and self-discipline. With a more modern approach to the treatment of depression, many people have been taught how to deal with mental illness by making changes in their lifestyle, by exercising, taking medication, or learning how to avoid the triggers that cause depression. Talk therapy and some forms of alternative medicine such as biofeedback and acupuncture have been used successfully. In fact, I am repeatedly surprised to find how many people I know who have been under treatment and managed their depression for a long time without any outward signs of problems.

Some Types of Depressive Illness

- Major depression may cause periods of sadness, emotional pain and misery. When severe, it can have an effect on how one functions at home or at work. Sleeping, eating, decision making, even the ability to get out of bed in the morning all become too hard to do. Some people may talk of suicide.
- Seasonal Affective Disorder, SAD, is a form of depression, which occurs in fall or winter when days are shorter and less sunny and usually disappears in spring and summer.
- Manic-depressive Illness, (bipolar disorder) alternates major lows or depression with inappropriate highs. During manic episodes a person can become overly active, voluble, euphoric and/or irritable and sensitive.

Resource

This is a very personal account of how bipolar disorder affects a person and those around her. It is sensitively written and helps one understand the puzzling behavior of a person with this disease.

An Unquiet Mind
By Kay Redfield Jamison—Random House Trade Paperbacks—
ISBN 0 679 44374

Possible Causes

- Family history may indicate a predisposition to depression although it is not a certainty that one will suffer from it. The risk is somewhat higher for those with bipolar disorder.
- Biochemical factors are indicated and being studied as possible causes.
- Life stressors such as the death of a loved one, chronic illness, financial problems, or moving from a long-time home can be triggers for depression.
- Psychosocial patterns established in childhood or adolescence such as low self-esteem, pessimism, or a feeling of no control over one's life can make someone more susceptible to depression in later years.
- Medication taken for another condition may cause depression as a side effect.

Signs to Look For

A person suffering from depression may give signals that are confusing and difficult to perceive. Having the insight to know when we ourselves may need help is even more difficult. Not all characteristics listed below will fit everyone who is depressed, but any one of them or a combination of several, which last for two weeks or longer indicate a need to seek help.

- Lack of interest in things previously enjoyed.
- Speaking softly, slowly, almost like a robot with little expression
- Being withdrawn, unwillingness to participate in conversations
- Sluggishness, sleeping more than usual, a reluctance or inability to get out of bed or get dressed.
- Inability to make even the smallest decisions, like brushing teeth or eating
- Persistent insomnia or sleep disruption with frequent awakenings and being unable to go back to sleep again

- A quick temper and low frustration level. Small problems are relived over and over again and can't be let go.
- Low self-esteem makes a person suspicious and quick to take offense.
- Abuse of alcohol, a depressant itself, in an attempt to forget feelings of inadequacy, self-loathing and hopelessness.
- Anxiety or panic attacks when the mind constantly recycles unreasonable thoughts and fears.
- Speaking of a plan for suicide or expressing a desire "to be gone from this world".
- A sudden loss or gain of weight indicating no interest in food or the need to eat all the time.
- Short-term memory loss and confusion.
- Loss of interest in sex.

Although symptoms for the depressive phase of the bipolar patient are much the same as those above, the manic phase brings on the following exaggeration of what could be called personality traits;

- Always being the life of the party or the comedian. Talking a mile a minute, constantly joking, moving around and searching for new things to do.
- Being a workaholic. Loading up the calendar as a distraction from how badly one feels. Working selflessly for others with no regard for personal priorities.
- Perfectionism that causes one to suffer over every detail, be highly critical and impossible to satisfy.

Where and How to Get Help

The first step, particularly for the person who may be reluctant to consult a psychiatrist, is to have a complete physical by a primary care physician to ensure that problems are not from the effect of medications being taken or a previously unidentified health condition. The doctor should pay particular attention to diet and nutritional status because a deficiency in some vitamins or minerals can be a cause of depression.

Often one is encouraged to seek treatment by a family member who has noticed that there are increasing signs of sadness or illness. I have been in that position and have been frustrated that the doctor did not see what I saw. My consultant suggested the reason why this happens is that a doctor makes a diagnosis by evaluating a "snapshot" of the patient during a short consultation when a "movie", or many impressions would give a much fuller picture. The next time I took my friend to the doctor, I asked if she would mind if I shared my observations of her symptoms during the visit. I took in a written list of behaviors and problems, which had been troubling her over a period of time and which the doctor could then use to diagnose her illness. To someone skilled in this type of diagnostic work another source of information can be invaluable.

Although a primary care doctor can prescribe anti-depressant medication, the best approach is to deal with the whole illness, not just the symptoms. Seeking help from one who is skilled in resolving life's issues, such as a spiritual advisor, social worker or psychiatrist can be effective. Life will always be full of ups and downs and even tragedies, but getting help for depression when the problems seem overwhelming makes just as much sense as seeing a physician when we have broken a leg. Keep in mind that it may take two or three tries before finding the most effective therapist.

Treatment Options

- Anti-depressants are often given to relieve physical symptoms, usually for a period of months and then a maintenance dose may be prescribed for a longer time if necessary. Many medications do not take effect for weeks until a proper level is reached in the body so regular monitoring including, in some cases regular blood checks, is required to minimize side effects. (**Note:** A physician,

pharmacist or nutritionist should check to be sure that medications taken for other conditions, including over the counter, vitamins and food supplements do not interact negatively with the antidepressant)
- Psychotherapy with a trained therapist may help someone gain insight into problems and to find ways to solve them.
- Cognitive Therapy helps one to learn how to deal with the day-to-day effects of depression, anxiety or stress. This may be done by a psychologist or trained social worker.
- Electro-convulsive therapy, ECT, has been an effective treatment for people at high risk of suicide and for the older patient when drug therapy is ineffective or for those who are suffering physical debilitation due to other physical illness.
- Nutritional therapy, the prescribing of vitamin and mineral supplements, especially Vitamin B or folic acid, has been shown to be of great value for some.
- Exercise used in conjunction with the above treatments may be prescribed to encourage recovery.
- Therapy using light that has the full wavelength of natural light has been used successfully for people with Seasonal Affective Disorder, SAD.
- Alternative or integrative medicine such as acupuncture, biofeedback, meditation, massage therapy, etc., in addition to traditional therapy should not be overlooked.

Beware "Contagious" Depression

Living with or being close to someone who is depressed can be emotionally draining. I know from personal experience that, even though understanding the disorder intellectually, it is difficult not to react to the mood and behavior changes experienced by a person suffering from depression. People who study such problems find that family members and caregivers of someone who is depressed will sometimes end up suffering some of the same symptoms. Even with the greatest of understanding, personal relationships can become so troubled that everyone involved could do with support.

The period leading up to diagnosis and subsequent treatment can be one of increasing tension and disruption of regular family relationships. Even after problems are identified as arising from a medical or emotional condition, recovery can take a long time and be in increments too small to be recognized. Some medications take weeks to reach an effective level in the body and, just as the condition did not become severe overnight, recovery may not be immediate.

One of the frustrating things about being intimately involved with depression is that both the sufferer and the supporter sometimes feel as though depression is something they should be able to handle without resorting to professional help or medication. The reasons for depression are so complex that, although it may be possible to temporarily ease tensions resulting from the down times, the most promising approach comes from professionals skilled in this field. When depression is combined with the fear of growing old, it becomes even more complicated and needs to be resolved. Getting someone to face up to the fact that the pain they are feeling is indeed a serious medical problem, can be the most difficult part of the whole equation.

> *A friend called me in tears to tell me of her experiences helping her mother who lived nearby and who was becoming increasingly needy as her depression and dementia deepened. She said, "I feel more and more isolated from my own family and friends because I don't dare leave her alone for longer than a few moments. She used to be such an active woman who had her own business and a thousand other interests. Now, I can't get her to go to the doctor or eat unless I am there with her and she refuses to see any of her old friends. I have taken more days off from work than I should and my husband, although sympathetic, is increasingly resentful of my absences. Sometimes, I don't want to get out of bed to face my mother's problems because I can't get her to face her own."*

Survival Techniques

- Take control of what seems to be an insoluble problem by learning about symptoms and treatment options.
- Miracles don't just happen. For some people, depression is an ongoing battle lasting for many years, even a lifetime, but in many cases it can be kept under control with medication and/or therapy.
- The supporter or caregiver's health is just as important. Caring for someone with depression is not an easy job. Getting help for one's-self when it is needed directly affects the health and well-being of the person being helped.
- Writing in a daily journal is something I found to be a great comfort and continue to use to this day when trying to understand the problems of someone with bipolar disorder. In it I record my frustrations and my own pain when things seem most discouraging. I have written letters to the person with whom I was having trouble relating but never mailed them and it helped a lot. This method expresses the sadness and even anger in a way that can hurt no one and on rereading in a calmer moment can lead to a more objective view of what is happening. Because the journal is so personal, it can be judgmental or as unreasonable as my emotions make it.

Staying the Course. Helping Someone to Continue Medication When They Don't Think They Need It.

Suffering with someone who is struggling with depression is bad enough but it is particularly disheartening when a loved one reaches a level of wellness and then abandons treatment against the doctor's advice because things seem so much better and they figure they don't need it any more. This happens most frequently with the bipolar patient. Seeing signs of the illness reassert themselves after a period of relative stability is difficult to accept but this behavior is by no means unusual. Often it is the reality that someone must take medication forever that causes him or her to stop taking it. In doing research for this chapter, I was given a tip by someone skilled in this field. She suggested that one make a contract with the person to take the medication for a period of time like a month, or a year and then reevaluate and renegotiate a new contract at the end of that time. It has not worked for us but it might for others.

Note: Remember that body needs change as weight and age change so if one is taking medication over a long period of time remind the prescribing doctor of those changes.

Resource

I found this book to be very helpful in identifying symptoms, understanding depression, its treatment and its effect on family members. A "must read" if suspecting that a loved one is depressed but not able to get him or her to treatment.
For information on depression in the elderly;
>*When Someone You Love is Depressed: How to help Your Loved One Without Losing Yourself*
>Aura Epstein Risen and Xavier Francisco Amateur—The Free Press—
>ISBN 0 684 82407 8

>American Assoc. for Geriatric Psychiatry, 7910 Woodmont Avenue, Bethesda, MD, 20814—*www.aagpgpa.org*
>National Depressive and Manic-Depressive Assoc.—*800 826-3632—www.ndma.org*

To get information on mental health issues or order publications about them call the following or go to the Website.
>Available from the US Department of Health and Human Services—800 421-4211—*www.hhs.gov*

This is a wonderful Website for caregivers and includes a good treatise on how to care for someone who is depressed.
>*www.ec-online.net*

When Someone Threatens to Take his or her own Life

From the information I have found on the subject, it is clear that any threat of suicide should be taken seriously. Older people, those from 65 to 85, are at particular risk of unrecognized and untreated mental illness, which is held as a leading cause of most cases of suicide in the elderly. Another fact that surprised me is that 20% of those people had seen their primary care physician the very day they took their own lives and 70% within a month of that event. Many doctors do not recognize symptoms of depression or suicidal tendencies thus it is friends and relatives who are most apt to see signs that things are not going well and will hopefully be able to steer someone who is severely depressed to the help they need. A doctor trained in geriatric medicine, either as a general practitioner, a specialist or a psychiatrist can recognize signs in the elderly that others miss. There are suicide hot lines and organizations to go to for referral and information on suicide prevention.

Persons who are determined to take their own lives will in many cases be successful. We can try to do everything we can to help but at the end of the day, if an attempt at suicide is successful, we need to tell ourselves that it was a decision and course we probably could not have changed.

RESOURCE

This national hot line will connect one with local crisis services.
    Suicide Hot Line—800 SUICIDE

National Mental Health Association—800 969-6642—*www.nmha.org*
American Foundation for Suicide Prevention—888 333-2377—*www.afsp.org*

Memory Doesn't Have To Be The First Thing To Go

Most of us suspect that aging will cause some memory impairment. Having seen elderly relatives and friends who have suffered from dementia or Alzheimer's disease, we sometimes worry needlessly that we are forgetting more and more things ourselves and that the same fate may be around the corner for us.

Researchers Confirm that Brainpower in Healthy People does not Decrease because of Advancing Age

The healthy brain never loses its capacity to learn and absorb new information. In fact recent research shows that a healthy person continues to grow brain cells throughout life. Although there are some things which are easier to learn and absorb at an early age such as language, there are many people of 80, 90 and 100 years who are alert and have lively, inquiring minds. The clear implication is that brain function becomes impaired more as a result of disease, medication or decreased use of the brain resulting from isolation than as a direct result of aging. Studies have proven that each of us can take an active role in staying mentally agile by being physically, socially and intellectually alert.

Understand about Normal Memory Loss

- Remembering takes longer with age because there's more information to sift through. I prefer to think of my brain as an aged computer. It does not process information as quickly as I would like because it is overloaded with information but it can access almost anything if I give it time.
- Undetected hearing problems play a large part in the way new information is recorded and stored. There are many people who have hearing loss. They may not appear deaf but they do not hear words properly and are confused because of it. Asking for things to be repeated all the time causes embarrassment so many people hope they heard it right and move on, often with a mistaken impression.
- Inadequate nutrition could cause a decrease in attentiveness and increase in confusion; therefore information may not be retained well.

- Stress induced memory loss can occur at any age. There are few of us who have not forgotten a luncheon date, walked into a room and couldn't remember what we were looking for or lost track of a name only minutes after being introduced. These are normal lapses, not to be confused with serious and persistent memory loss and often occur because there are too many things going on at once, or perhaps because we didn't pay as much attention as we should have. An example; you can't find the car keys for the umpteenth time. That's just not keeping in mind where you left them. The real problem is when you can't remember what they are used for.
- Most experts in the field will tell us, *USE IT OR LOSE IT!* One specialist likens memory to a muscle of the mind. Exercise will keep it fit, practice will increase its skill.

Some Useful Hints

- When meeting a new person, repeat the name aloud then make a point of introducing that person to someone else to reinforce the memory.
- Pay better attention! Repeat instructions back to the doctor to be sure they are clear and complete.
- Do calisthenics for the brain frequently. "Brain teasers", crossword word puzzles, geography quizzes, poetry memorization all involve processing and retaining information. Participate in neighborhood organizations, attend lecture groups, volunteer for political campaigns and/or learn how to use a computer.
- Keep up social and intellectual interaction with all ages, younger and older. Friends' lives tend to march on without us if social invitations are avoided or a way is not found to see them on a regular basis. There is increasing evidence that people who are outgoing, open minded; creative and curious tend to retain better memory skills.

Develop the habit of keeping lists, writing notes and dating them. Keep paper and pencil by the phone, record appointments in a calendar as they are made. Use a steno pad to record decisions made, projects to do, things to pick up at the store then cross them out as they are done.

- Write daily appointments on a dated 3x5 card as a way to keep from forgetting all the details of a busy day, and put it where it can be referred to when needed. Draw a line through each appointment or project completed.
- Purchase a birthday calendar, fill it out and hang it on the refrigerator or the inside of the bathroom door. That way it will be seen several times a day.
- Get in the habit of leaving eyeglasses, car and house keys in the same place in rooms most frequented. I have wasted so many hours looking for all of these items that this is a lifesaver for me.
- Take a memory course.
- Keep a daily journal. Get in the habit of writing things to do or appointments to keep in one place. Date the entries.
- Establishing these habits before problems appear can give anyone confidence to face complications of a busy life for years to come even if memory loss is not acute.

Resource

I have scanned this book but found it to be well written and set up. It is a good reference for many problems found in aging and explains the relationship of good health of the body to that of the brain.

Keep Your Brain Young The Complete Guide to Physical and Emotional Health and Longevity
By Guy McKhann, M.D. and Marilyn Albert, PhD—John Wiley & Sons, 2002—ISBN 0-471-40792-5

For an interesting and useful series of memory exercises contact this organization and request this special bulletin.

United Seniors Health Cooperative—Special Report 49—202 479 1200

When Memory Loss becomes too Serious to Ignore

Get help from the experts when there are signs that serious cognitive deficits are getting in the way of coping with daily life. Memory loss can be caused by so many factors that if the problems become persistent and worrisome they should be checked by a doctor to rule out such things as depression, diet deficiencies, medication, stroke or other physiological conditions. Ask for a referral to a geriatric or neuro-psychiatric specialist if the primary physician is not familiar with requirements and treatment of the elderly.

There are many of us in mid-life who have mumbled about memory loss or Alzheimer's to cover the embarrassment of forgetting something, but there is not one of us who hasn't had a thought now and then that such a fate would be devastating. It is for this reason that we should make ourselves familiar with some other forms of cognitive failure.

Dementia Syndrome

The clinical description of dementia is that it is a global decline in intellectual functioning of sufficient severity to impair social or occupational functioning while in a clear state of consciousness; i.e. not caused by coma, etc. More simply the dictionary defines dementia as a loss or impairment of mental powers due to organic causes. We have seen that dementia is characterized by confusion, memory loss and disorientation, and interferes with a person's ability to carry out daily activities. To remind, true dementia is irreversible but is not an inevitable part of growing older.

Many people, as they reach middle age and beyond, harbor a fear of dementia far exceeding the reasonable chances of their falling victim to it. A consultant from the Neuropsychiatry and Memory Clinic at Johns Hopkins put it into perspective for me. 6% of Americans over the age of 65 suffer from some form of dementia. *Of that 6%,* 20% have what is known as vascular dementia caused by tiny strokes invisible to the observer, 20% show signs of dementia because of diseases such as Parkinson's, Huntington's Disease, Multiple Sclerosis, etc., 10% have treatable conditions mimicking dementia as listed below, and 50% of that original 6%, suffer from Alzheimer's Disease. Statistics can be used to back up any thesis . . . it is a good idea to know the whole picture before accepting what you have read.

Pseudodementia

Diagnosing and treating mental illness and emotional disorders is a complex process requiring even more specialized knowledge if the patient is elderly. Someone may become forgetful, disoriented, or confused because of a quickly reversible condition caused by drug interaction or overdose, poor diet, disease, and/or some chronic physical illnesses.

Some of the factors causing the problem

Drugs

Because metabolism slows with age, drugs can stay in the body longer and reach toxic levels more quickly, a fact doctors trained in geriatric medicine and certified nutritionists usually recognize. A person suffering from dementia may not be able to give an accurate accounting of the medications being taken, including over the counter remedies thus confusion may add to the problem of overdosing. A doctor may prescribe medication without having a full picture of all the factors causing the symptoms of dementia therefore it is critical to diagnosis to have an accurate accounting of all medications being taken.

Alcoholic beverages may be compounding the toxic effects of drugs causing confusion, mood changes and other symptoms of dementia. Alcoholism or high consumption of alcohol with its "empty" calories can depress appetite for nutritious foods leading to a form of malnutrition, which can also lead to dementia. Alcohol depletes B vitamins, zinc and other nutrients essential to the maintenance of brain function.

Poor Nutrition

The brain needs a steady supply of proper nutrients therefore poor eating habits caused by sore gums and teeth, or problems with digestion, can have an effect on the way the brain works. Vitamins and minerals, such as lithium and folate, play a particularly important role in physical and emotional health. Drinking enough water to increase blood volume to the brain, eating regular, nutritional meals and the addition of nutritional supplements, if needed are vital for good mental and physical health.

In some people, acid release in the stomach could be so low from the use of antacids that nutrients, which require an acid environment for availability, are not extracted from food. If this situation continues it is possible to develop nutritional deficiencies causing symptoms, appearing to be dementia. Anyone taking antacids on a regular basis for digestive upset should ask someone skilled in the field of nutrition for an evaluation.

Diseases of the Heart and Lung

Lack of oxygen can affect the brain and behavior. When the systems that carry oxygen to the brain are impaired, as in a stroke or series of them, (Multi—infarct dementia) symptoms of dementia may result. Chronic high blood pressure can be another factor.

Diseases of the Adrenal, Thyroid, Pituitary or other Glands

Diabetes, particularly in the elderly can be a problem as the affected glands help regulate emotions, perceptions, memory and thought processes. When they are not working properly, they can also cause symptoms of dementia.

Clinical Depression

Unexplained memory loss, or the ability to concentrate, confusion and disorientation are only some of the symptoms of depression that can mimic dementia.

Deafness

Being able to hear what people are saying is central to

understanding, to retaining knowledge and being able to do the things we need to do daily, such as going to the store or having conversations on the phone.

> *Until recently, a friend was actively involved in running a small business and had been a welcome addition to any social gathering, but it was noticed that he was becoming more and more withdrawn. He fumbled answers to questions, confused simple instructions in the household and caused most of his friends to assume that he was sliding into a form of dementia. It was finally understood that he was becoming increasingly deaf and couldn't face having to accept such a loss or the possibility of having to wear a hearing aid.*

Multi-Infarct Dementia

Sometimes called vascular dementia, this is a condition of the brain caused by many little strokes. The blockage of a blood vessel in the brain restricts the flow of blood to the brain and destroys brain tissue by cutting off oxygen and nutrients to that area. These small strokes cause an inability to function in various ways thus displaying symptoms of multi-infarct dementia. A person suffering such strokes can show marked improvement for a short time and then abrupt changes in mental ability as more small strokes occur. This type of dementia is more common in late life and particularly in those with high blood pressure and diabetes.

Alzheimer's Disease, (AD)

The fourth leading cause of death in the US, AD can strike in the early middle years, (called early onset) but is found most often later in life. AD is a progressive, degenerative disease that causes brain cells to die. At the moment there is no known cause, no definite way to diagnose AD until after death and no cure, although there are many promising studies being done. It often begins in the part of the brain controlling short-term memory and progresses to affect one's ability to reason and perform routine tasks. The disease takes different forms in each individual and can take 8 to 20 years to run its course. The good news is that as a larger population is growing older, there is more attention being focused on this disease. Hopeful avenues are being explored for diagnosis and understanding of the causes of AD leading to a possible cure. There are also encouraging results of preliminary studies on new medications, vitamin and estrogen therapy with insurance companies and Medicare being more willing to reimburse for them as the effectiveness of such treatments allow patients to live independently longer.

Support services for patients and their families, including adult day care facilities, ID bracelets for those who may wander from home, respite care arrangements for the caregiver, are easier to find than they were a few years ago. Assisted living facilities, which specialize in treating and caring for the AD or dementia syndrome patient are an intermediate alternative to a nursing home.

Some Clues to Look For

- Short-term memory loss. When asking a question, the person may not remember having asked it several times already. Nutrition suffers because he cannot remember if he has eaten or not. Family members become impatient because things have been forgotten, which were discussed yesterday or even this morning.
- Uncharacteristic trouble handling money, and working with numbers. Paying bills and keeping simple accounts becomes confusing.
- Disorientation. Not knowing what day it is, having trouble organizing daily activities, or understanding what has just been read is a clue that something is wrong. This is the extreme and repeated incidence rather than the episodic events we all suffer now and then.
- Difficulty in communicating, not being able to find the right word, being unable to finish thoughts or to follow directions are also signs of problems.

- Mild personality changes appear such as increased lack of energy and contact with friends.
- Irritability, being argumentative, and combative, if it is not part of regular behavior should be another signal that something is wrong.
- Losing the way when going to or from a familiar destination, or feeling lost in well-known surroundings may happen with increasing frequency.

What to Do Now

This section of the chapter is equally as important for the person who is worried about the possibility of dementia herself as it is for someone who cares for a loved one showing such signs.

- The first step is diagnosis. Sort out what the symptoms are, and seek help from an expert in geriatric or neuropsychiatric medicine. The sooner a proper work-up is done the sooner problems can be resolved and a person can begin to take control of the effort to retain cognitive function as long as possible. In our experiences with the Neuropsychiatry and Memory Clinic at Johns Hopkins Hospital in Baltimore, I have been impressed with the positive attitude of everyone we consulted. The first myth they dispelled was that AD is an untreatable condition. There are four areas of treatment this facility specifies;

    - Treat the disease
    - Treat the symptoms
    - Support the patient
    - Support the family

Positive diagnosis of AD is possible only after death at this time, but most specialists can rule out other causes by a process of elimination. A patient going to a clinic or doctor experienced in evaluating cognitive disorders usually starts with asking for a medical history and then probably neuro-psychological tests will be administered to check memory, problem solving ability and language skills. Remember that all of us have had problems with some or all of the symptoms of AD now and then. It is when these problems become persistent that we need to seek help for someone we care for or for ourselves. Also, keep in mind that for those of us who are dyslexics, spatial, numerical and spelling testing may give an inappropriate result so we should mention that fact to the testing technician.

Resource

This is without a doubt the best book I have read on the subject and the most sympathetic explanation of the whole process of Alzheimer's disease. The author brings an historical perspective to the disease at the same time as making the scientific information clear and easy to read. This is a must for anyone with any connection to dementia or Alzheimer's disease. For the caregiver, it gives invaluable support and understanding.

The Forgetting Alzheimer's: Portrait of an Epidemic
By David Shenk—Doubleday—2001—ISBN 0-385-49837-3

Do What it takes to Stay Independent as Long as Possible

While doing research for this book, I found a lot of information in libraries and bookstores for the caregiver of the AD patient but very little on assisting the person diagnosed with AD to help himself. Recently, mainstream organizations such as AARP have publicized information on new drugs that slow the effects of AD and strategies designed to keep a patient independent and functioning well for a much longer period of time than had been supposed before. To begin to take control of a life, which seems to be slipping away, and to slow down the effects of the disease by early medical intervention and taking steps in the first stages of the disease to deal with daily aggravations and losses is to be given hope. I read a book called *Living in the Labyrinth,* written by a woman who suffered early onset AD. Her confusion and distress was increased by the anger and frustration of those closest to her who could not understand why she kept getting lost or couldn't complete simple transactions any more. It was her ability to think up ways to triumph over those obstacles, which gives hope for others diagnosed with AD.

Resource

I found this book so full of hope and ability to cope with increasing difficulties living a normal life that I believe anyone having memory problems ought to read it.
Living in the Labyrinth—A Personal Journey Through the Maze of Alzheimer's
By Diana Friel McGowin—Delta Publishing 1994—ISBN: 0-385-3138-7

The progression of symptoms can be very slow with periods of relative stability lasting for several years. There are things one can do to move from fear through denial into acceptance by first seeing a doctor and being evaluated in the early stages. Once a positive diagnosis is made, compensating for skills lost with strategies listed below to stay independent as long as possible is a next step. Use those strategies to make realistic plans for care knowing that the disease will inevitably progress. Stimulating social contact, pushing oneself to learn new things, devising shortcuts, taking medication, which holds off the effects of AD for a period of time, making the choice to keep control of life as long as possible has been proven to delay onset of the worst effects of dementia and Alzheimer's.

Life with a diagnosis of AD is not entirely without hope, particularly as progress is being made on its treatment and diagnosis. One does not just wake up one morning totally incapacitated. Problems with memory and cognitive function, if they are caused by AD, come slowly and over a prolonged period of time in most cases therefore a willingness to accept challenges and define the battleground may be the most effective weapons to delay the worst effects of the disease.

- Become a problem solver in the effort to keep a "plan for independence" flexible and be able to respond to changing needs. If the old way of doing things does not work, find shortcuts, simplify tasks and use memory aids to keep track of things slipping by.
- Build a support system into any planning. Fighting the effects of a disease like AD is a lonely battle. At the same time, one of the greatest frustrations for loved ones is that they would like to help but haven't any idea how to do so. Once a diagnosis has been made, coming up with a plan for friends and relatives to be part of the solution is a key to long term well being. Anyone living alone can contact a chapter of the Alzheimer's Association to find a support group, meet with a social worker to see what options are for the future, and put in place appropriate steps for daily living.
- Consult an attorney. Execute a Durable Power of Attorney, a Health Care Power of Attorney, a Living Will and write your will. In other words, put your financial affairs in order.
- Become an expert on the disease. Learn about experimental programs and new treatments, the best clinics, the best programs.
- Staying safe and healthy as long as possible is the objective therefore knowing what to expect during the course of the disease is important. Involving oneself in the "coping" process helps to hold off the feeling of lack of control characteristic of increasing dementia. Joining a support group of early stage AD patients helps one strategize his or her own approach to dealing with life.
- Resist the temptation to compare the person you are now as an AD patient to the one you once were. Help friends and family to do the same thing. Do not forget that AD is a progressive disease so that strategies that work today will have to be changed and adjusted as the need arises.

- Start simplifying life. Routine daily living, keeping clean, eating well, grocery shopping, the taking of medications, bill paying and house maintenance, may be difficult enough when in the best of health, but now is the time to phase in a helping system for these tasks, which can escalate as need dictates.
- Do not neglect the care and feeding of family relationships and social contacts. Social stimulation has been proven to be a way to slow the progression of the disease. Arrange a daily telephone visit with a close friend or family member who is aware of the "plan for independence" so they can be a part of the effort.
- Knowing what day it is. Establish the habit of using the daily newspaper as a reference by circling the day and date on the calendar the moment the paper is brought into the house. Put a small blackboard in a prominent place where a lot of time is spent. The date can be noted and erased each day.
- Stay interested in the outside world. Find an article of interest, write down a summary of the facts, date it and then call a friend and discuss it. Do the same with magazines or periodicals or books. This is a great way for friends to stay involved.
- Open the mail in the same room and place every day. Get three boxes and label them BILLS, PERSONAL, and JUNK MAIL. Before anything is thrown away, someone who is part of the support system should check to see that nothing vital is overlooked.
- Keep a calendar by the phone used most frequently and tie it securely so that it cannot be removed. Place notepads by each phone with a good supply of pens or pencils and learn to enter the date beside each entry. Buy a birthday calendar, fill it out and then post it on the refrigerator or bathroom door. This is one more way to stay a part of other people's lives.
- Establish a defense system for door-to-door salesmen and telephone solicitors. Get a small card or paper and tape it

by each phone to be referred to when telemarketers call saying;
- "THANK YOU FOR YOUR CALL BUT I NEVER SUPPORT ORGANIZATIONS SOLICITING OVER THE PHONE."
- Take care of door-to-door salesmen the same way. Place a sign outside the front door saying;
- "I NEVER PURCHASE ITEMS SOLD AT MY DOOR"
- The door should never be opened to strangers and if salesmen persist put another sign by the inside the front door saying the same thing so it can be repeated through the closed door.
- Have an inventory taken of small, high value, personal items in the house, (jewelry, coins, stamp collections, family memorabilia, etc.) and then see that they are put in a safe place with a copy of the inventory to a lawyer or trusted friend. This is to assure that nothing gets lost or stolen if the assistance of hired caretakers is needed in the future.
- Arrange for a bill paying service so that a system of checks, balances and oversight can be installed. Personal Information files should be accessible to a lawyer and a designated relative or friend. Have income checks direct deposited, and statements balanced. Name someone else to check the figures periodically to ensure that no mistakes or fraud take place. "Carbonless checks" are a great aid for keeping track of every check written and would assist the person doing the statements to keep the figures straight until writing checks oneself is no longer feasible.
- Keep memories fresh by starting an album of family pictures and labeling them. Add theater stubs and postcards of places visited. Label and date everything then go back and refer to it frequently. Simplify getting from here to there with easy to read maps of destinations often traveled to. One reference suggested having someone draw separate maps, which can be kept in clear plastic holders showing how to get to the supermarket, library, gas station, etc. with the way home on the reverse side. Always mark the direction of one-way

streets and have the home address and perhaps even the phone number of a friend or relative printed on each page.
- An ID bracelet with address and phone number of the patient should always be worn for the time when disorientation is complete and the person has no idea how to get home.

Being a Caregiver For the AD Patient

Many who have seen elderly friends and relatives as they gradually lost that sense of self, which defined who and what they were, know the despair that cannot be compared to any other. Helping the person being cared for by using some of the strategies above can slow the effects of AD but not stop them. There is also much we must do for ourselves, as caregivers to remain strong during what can be a draining and exhausting process.

Strategies

- Join a support group, get information from the experts and avoid listening to horror stories.
- Good health for the caregiver is as important as for the patient. Being tired or sick will help no one. Periodic respite care through local agencies or an adult day care center if it becomes appropriate is sometimes necessary.
- Accept the possibility that at times each of us will be discouraged; feel frustrated, overburdened and often guilty about feeling that way.
- There may be a time when full time care and perhaps a move to a nursing facility is required because providing the necessary specialized care becomes too difficult. We found this moment to be very emotional when we were caregivers and we needed reinforcement from other family members that such a decision had to be made. There are facilities catering to the AD patient, some of them very good.
- Help family members to be comfortable with the AD patient, particularly children and grandchildren, as both

caregiver and patient need to remain part of the world. Large crowds may be too confusing but small gatherings can be comforting. Children often become shy and increasingly uncomfortable as they sense that there is something wrong with a person who is ill. One friend told of helping her children relate to her mother who was becoming increasingly forgetful by asking them to do a memory book for and with her. When they visited her they added pages to the book and had something to talk about.

- Keep current with new treatments and new ideas for helping the AD patient retain as much memory as possible.
- One innovation tried by Dr. Gene D. Cohen of George Washington University Hospital Medical School was to see whether a biographical video of the patient narrated by a family member would stimulate "pockets of memory" and help interaction with family members. The reaction has exceeded researcher's expectations. It is a somewhat complicated process using a video camera but there might be students in film classes or art schools or local professionals who could put such a video together.

Resource

This is considered the definitive handbook on helping the person with dementia of any kind.

The 36-Hour Day, A Family Guide To Caring For Persons With Alzheimer's Disease, Related Dementing Illness and Memory Loss in Later Life
By Nancy L. Mace, MA and Peter V. Rabins, MD, MPH—Warner Books—2001

- Safety-proof the house. A social worker can help give guidelines for this process.
- Establish a simple routine for daily living and personal hygiene. Change is very unsettling.
- Assign tasks one at a time and with simple, one step

instructions. Praise for success goes a long way toward encouraging self-sufficiency whereas criticism and arguing can increase agitation.
- Ask questions so they can be answered with a yes or no.
- Find the most effective way to share information with the doctor on changes in health or behavior. Often a patient with AD can put on his or her best behavior thus masking real problems.
- Keep expectations realistic by understanding the nature of progression of the effects of AD. It is difficult to know what part of the brain is being affected today and what will cause problems tomorrow. Sometimes there will be flashes of better functioning and then in a very short time more loss.
- Plan to include some days off, (respite care). It gives the patient a chance to get used to having someone else in the home for short periods of time or going to a day-care facility before a more full time option is needed. More importantly it is a time for the caregiver to count on for him or herself.
- When frustration becomes unbearable, practice deep breathing exercises to help bring yourself some equilibrium.
- If the disease has progressed to the point that communication is difficult to impossible, remind doctors treating the patient for chronic conditions like arthritis or such things as a broken hip, that just because a person can't communicate about how much pain they are in, it does not mean they should not be treated just as aggressively for discomfort as any other person. I am heartened to read that some doctors will opt for pain amelioration in the end stages of AD rather than putting someone through surgery when his or her quality of life is already limited.

Medicare Rules on Early Treatment for AD

In the spring of 2002, a ruling was made that Medicare patients can apply for reimbursement of therapy and treatment costs of early AD. Because of advances in early diagnosis of AD and the development of drugs that can slow its effects it has been decided that such expenditure actually saves money in the long run due to the fact that people are able to stay independent far longer than had once been the case. The criteria are the same as with any other Medicare claim and that is that the treatment should be judged appropriate for the condition.

Resource

This group can put one in contact with support groups for people in every stage of AD. They also have the latest information on hopes for cure as well as care giving assistance.

The Alzheimer's Association
PO Box 5675 DEPT.P
Chicago, Illinois 60680—800 272-3900

www.alz.org

Alzheimer's Disease Education and Referral (ADEAR) Center
PO Box 8250
Silver Spring, MD 20907-8250—800 438-4380

www.alzheimers.org

Once again, AARP has a publication, which could be of help for the caregiver of an AD patient.

Ask for: "Steps to Success: Decisions about Help at Home for Alzheimer's Caregivers—D17623

"Nurturing a Family Partnership: Alzheimer's Home Care Aide's Guide—D17624

AARP Fulfillment (EEO1529
601 E ST NW
Washington, DC 20049

CHAPTER SEVEN

Turning Worry About The Future Into A Positive Exercise

Assuming that we have planned our financial resources to be sufficient to the end of our lives and that we have considered the possibility we may live to be 100 or more, we must also be certain that they are managed in such a way that they keep pace with the economic pressures placed upon them and unforeseen catastrophic events that could occur. We should know what our options are to get the greatest mileage we can from what we have already and to see our nest egg increase in order to respond to emergencies and unexpected financial needs. The way to do that is to consult the experts and to stay knowledgeable by periodic updates of our financial condition.

Bringing Adult Children Into the Equation

Making the transition from parent as unquestioned authority figure to parent as friend and almost equal does not come easily or overnight but is part of a process of drawing our children along with us as our needs and theirs change. Dynamics within the family are never static; therefore healthy relationships require adjustment, flexibility and trust. The rewards for making such an effort last for many lifetimes.

Letting our children know how we feel about the way we wish to be treated in a life-threatening situation and seeing that we have the proper legal means to assure that our wishes will be followed makes good sense. Being flexible and responsive to possible disabling factors in our lifestyle as they appear makes clear that we can make our own decisions about our limitations and indicates a desire to shield them from worry. It makes perfect sense to talk over these issues with our children or other close relatives before the possibility that illness or cognitive failure could thrust us into a situation where we are helpless to control the course of our lives or even how we wish to leave it.

As we see older people living to unheard of years, it is becoming increasingly clear that income and assets must last a lot longer than they used to. Keep in mind that a man age 65 can statistically expect to live to the age of 80 and a woman to age 84. Having reached 85 and still in good health, there is a good chance that a person will live into his or her nineties and even 100. The largest percentage of those people will be women. Financial experts, after taking into consideration inflation, rising health costs and even the possibility of having to care for one's parents or a disabled adult child, are predicting a person will need between 60% and 80% of pre-retirement income after retiring. How those assets are managed is the key to whether one can maintain fiscal independence as long as needed.

Deciding to have a financial strategy is only the first step. Periodic review of one's resources as life circumstances change, income levels fluctuate, or tax requirements are revised is an ongoing process. Planning ahead may not be fun, but in this complicated time, it must be done

Planning ahead is not just for those in early middle age. It is for anyone who wishes to be prepared for the unexpected. It is for couples and singles and parents with children. It is for the young and the not so young, the middle aged and the elderly. It is for those of modest circumstances as much as it is for the wealthy.

Planning ahead, aside from making perfect sense, is an act of generosity to those who love you and a gift to those you love.

A Sound Partnership Calls for Full Disclosure

I am in my sixties. Many women of my generation did not work outside the home after marriage. Our husbands managed the finances and took on the responsibility of seeing that resources would exceed longevity. When we were married, I thought independence meant having my own checkbook and autonomy over my daily schedule. Little did I know about the possibility that a husband could suddenly pass away or medical expenses could deplete what a couple had planned for their retirement. The limit of my understanding of financial matters was the advice my mother gave me when we married;

- Have a checking account in your own name because you should never have to explain every item needed or wanted if it falls within available resources.
- A good marriage is built on trust but we should both know about all our financial obligations, income and investments. It wasn't until I was in my 50's that I heeded this advice.

If a spouse should suddenly die or divorce sever a relationship, having an account in one's own name may be the only way to access funds before an estate is settled. We should know what funds can be drawn on in an emergency and before legal necessities are completed.

Each of us must become knowledgeable about our own financial affairs. No matter how much faith we place in spouse, bank or accountant to manage them we risk decisions being made in the future that might not be in our best long-term interests. I accept the premise that it is my responsibility to think through and express what I wish for my own life. If that is so then it is also my responsibility to know what we own and what we owe and whether we will be able to pay for medical care during a catastrophic or prolonged illness. Blind trust when it has to do with one's own future and financial security is a luxury no one can afford. Trust backed with knowledge and the ability to ask the right questions is an insurance policy against coming up short in our later years when we are our most vulnerable. Questioning long time arrangements is not easy but not inserting oneself early in the process could cause a rude awakening when a spouse dies or funds are needed in an emergency. I have actually seen what can happen when one partner, handling the finances for a couple, creates a devastating situation because cognitive failure went unsuspected for years. A trusted personal secretary looted a sizable fortune to satisfy a love of betting on horse racing and a bank, handling a family trust fund, took better care of itself than it did the beneficiaries leaving them with a diminished inheritance.

My contract with myself mandates that I become knowledgeable about our financial health, insurance plans, and probable taxes and that I take an active part in future decisions. I want to know what my income will be if my husband should die before me and whether he will be equally secure if I should go first. I want to become accustomed to the thought that I might have to sell assets to make ends meet long before I have to. The thought of losing him is traumatic enough. I want to have a plan in place if the worst should happen. Habits are hard to break for both of us and I fight the impulse to have my eyes glaze over when discussing or reading about such matters. I have to know the questions to ask our financial advisor but must also be able to express my concerns for the future in a way that we both can accept. This is not to imply that what he has done is not the best for both of us. It is to admit that I have been woefully ignorant of what could be crucial to our future. Tax laws and ways to avoid them are appearing with the speed of light. Medical costs are rising as fast as insurance plans can find ways to avoid paying for them. Most of us need help to plot our way through the maze.

Preparing for the Unthinkable—
Becoming Suddenly Single

I have seen what can happen when misplaced faith that everything will turn out well left a frail elderly woman with limited funds to lead her life in the way she wished to after her husband passed away. I have seen a person my own age lose her husband in less than a minute and have to learn how to manage a complex estate with trusts, business contracts and personal obligations practically overnight. Another friend realized too late that her husband had been losing his ability to manage their accounts for several years and by the time he was diagnosed with Alzheimer's Disease their funds were seriously depleted.

In most marriages, one person manages the finances. In a true partnership, both members should know about every part of that arrangement. The process of estate planning prepares people like me for the responsibilities of money management if my spouse should die before me. Death of a spouse can leave a person numb with grief and shock. There are certain financial decisions that must be done in a timely fashion after the death of a partner and if we have done our homework before that moment, we can save our energies for the grieving process.

- We should become knowledgeable about all investments, contracts, real estate and financial assets, liabilities, savings, trusts and wills that involve us in any way, *right now*. The surviving partner may be liable for more than he or she can afford in the event of sudden death.
- Make an appointment to see a financial advisor.
- Calculate what income will be if either spouse should die then make a list of what are fixed expenses like mortgages, medical insurance, food, travel, vacation needs, etc. Planning for a possible shortfall if there will be any and creating a strategy to accommodate the future could help ease a traumatic time.
- Find out ahead of time what decisions will have to be made

- about contracts, investments, bills, etc. and have a plan for downsizing if income is reduced.
- Joint accounts are not always accessible immediately after the death of one account holder. Know where you can get enough cash to make mortgage payments, pay bills, or just to pay living expenses.

Resource

This book makes it easy to become knowledgeable about what one needs to know about finances when planning to retire.
Ask for the up-dated edition.

You've Earned it, Don't Lose It: Mistakes You Can't Afford to Make When You Retire
By Suze Ormond—Newmarket Press—ISBN 1-55704-316-7

I have only scanned this but feel that if I can understand it, it should be useful for anyone. Important information.

Suddenly Single: Money Skills for Divorcees and Widows
By Kerry Hannon—John Wiley & Sons, 1998—ISBN 0-47 1243 116

Do Your Heirs a Favor.
Create a Personal Information File

My mother was a businesswoman who raised three children alone. She managed her finances well enough that she needed for nothing before her last illness and death. When she was no longer able to manage her own affairs, my sister and I paid the nurses and maintained the house acting on the faith that there would always be enough to see her through the crisis but without specific documentation. We didn't want to ask the questions and she kept her affairs very private. It made a difficult situation stressful. I wish she had made a list of her financial assets, and liabilities, and any other contracts or obligations to which we could refer as the need arose. I wish she had shared it with us. When it was our responsibility to clear out the house after she died, we spent untold hours trying to track down the necessary information on her financial affairs as we found passbooks from savings banks, safe deposit keys, vague mentions of contracts to pay and other financial items all over the house. It made the task of settling her estate very time consuming and required the use of highly paid lawyers to finally set everything straight.

When we depart this earth, our survivors must prove our entitlement to the benefits we have designated for them. Things such as birth and marriage certificates, military discharge or retirement papers, divorce decrees, and of course social security numbers must be readily available. The location of insurance policies, contracts, mortgage, bank accounts, safe deposit box keys and authorization, stocks and bonds, automobile ownership, need to be made accessible for the person trying to settle the estate. Each year, millions of dollars are lost to their rightful owners and heirs because banks and dividend-paying companies could not find them.

Invest the Time and Trouble
it takes to gather all the Information in One Place

Maintaining independence takes work and that includes accepting responsibility for seeing that those closest to us know what makes up our estate and how to find the documentation to access it.

- No one says it has to be done in one day. Finding the time to go through such a process may seem impossible, but apply the principle that if there is time for one hour of work, it puts one further along than before. Take a category at a time and proceed. There is a worksheet at the end of this book to help you. (See Appendix A) Update that list at least once a year, when you pay off a loan, incur additional debt for any reason or make any kind of personal loan.

- Now see that it is left where family or relatives can find it. One father we know has met with his children each time there was a major change in his financial holdings or planning. In this way they know that he has planned for the future and at the same time they can realistically evaluate what has been planned for them.

Resource

For those who are members of The Retired Officer's Association there is an excellent workbook that helps one organize and record all of this information.

Help your Surviving Spouse—Now!

MOAA Attn llE
201 N. Washington ST.
Alexandria, VA 22314-2539

www.moaa.org

Don't Become a Victim of Identity Theft

We have friends who have been through the unnerving experience of finding unexplained charges on their credit card although the card had not been out of their possession at any time. In checking with the credit card company they were warned that it sounded like a classic case of identity theft . . . and it was. On the advice of the credit card company they called the credit reporting bureau numbers they were given and found signs of more trouble there. It took them months of frustrating work to clear their name and accounts. In this day of internet purchasing and many organizations asking for one's Social Security number, it is relatively easy for someone to steal your identity and charge up huge amounts to your credit cards, open new ones in your name, empty your bank accounts and generally create havoc with your financial life. An article in The Washington Post said that on average, a victim spends $175 and 1000 hours to clear his or her name.

There are a number of things one can do to avoid such a trauma and some of them are just common sense. This is only a partial list but you can access the article I read with more information on the Internet.

- Ask for your credit report from the three listed in the Resource section below at least once a year. Keep in mind that negative information can remain on your credit report for 7 years unless it is corrected. Get a paper shredder and use it for anything that has any piece of personal identity on it. Forget about recycling until it's shredded for that reason.
- Don't leave any mail in your own mailbox to be picked up by the mailman, such as paid bills, orders for checks, insurance payments, etc. That cute little red flag is an irresistible signal to someone who wants your vital statistics. Pick up mail as soon after it is delivered as possible for the same reason.
- Have checks printed with first initial and last name because it is more difficult to use someone else's identity if they don't know the first name.
- Keep your Social Security number to yourself. Don't carry it with you and don't give it out to anyone unless they can prove a legal necessity to have it.
- Photocopy all the cards in your wallet, both back and front, the number of which have been reduced to a bare minimum, and stash them in a secure place at home. If your wallet gets stolen, the speed with which you get to your credit card companies and others is key to stopping what could be far more damage than just a big credit card bill. Often what will happen when someone has your credit card, they will open another account in your name but with another address so that you are not even aware that charges are being made against your name.
- If receiving a call purporting to do with credit information, ask for the name of the person calling and call them back using a number you look up yourself for verification.

What do I do Now?

The article lists a number of things to be done if suspicious that you are a victim of identity theft.

- Ask for a "fraud alert" to be placed on your name at the three credit reporting bureaus listed below. Do the same with the Social Security Administration. Once that step has been taken, a company or creditor must contact you before authorizing new credit.
- File a police report where the theft occurred. Our friend was told that this was key to future prosecution of anyone caught for the theft. If you think the mail was involved, notify the local postmaster.
- Notify your bank and change your PIN's.
- The FTC maintains a national clearinghouse for victims of identity theft. If you file an ID Theft Affidavit, it alerts companies and organizations that they may have fraudulent accounts in your name.

RESOURCE

Your credit report can be requested from these credit reporting bureaus.
    Equifax—800 685-1111—*www.equifax.com*
    Experian—888 397-3742—*www.experian.com*
    TransUnion—800 888-4213—*www.tuc.com*
    FTC's Identity Theft hotline—877 IDTHEFT
To order a copy of your Social Security Statement:
                        800 772-1213—*www.ssa.gov/*
This is considered an excellent resource.
    The Identity Theft Resource Center—858 693-7935—*www.idtheftcenter.org*

If Everything I Had Was Lost Today, Would I Know What was Gone?

I can hear you saying . . . she must be crazy. How many times does lightning strike anyway? I am indeed a world-class worrier but lightning struck twice one summer at the homes of two friends of ours. One lost everything in the house and the other almost everything. They both spent months trying to piece together what was gone and it was an exhausting, stressful process. One had recently done a complete inventory of things in the house, but was in the process of putting it on her computer therefore it burned up in the fire along with everything else. Both of them said that the most difficult problem, aside from the drudgery of filling out a million forms and the emotional pain of such a loss, was to recreate in their minds everything that was a part of their lives in each room. Homeowner's insurance rarely covers everything owned but having an inventory gives one the satisfaction that the biggest portion has been recovered.

- Just get started! Doing a complete inventory with appraisals and original sale prices takes a long time but this is another one of those things that doesn't have to be done all in one day, or month. One hour added to two and to three more eventually gets the job done.
- Ask an insurance company for an inventory sheet to make the notations more organized or find one in an office supply store, which may have a place for pictures to accompany items.
- Use a video, digital or still camera to help document what is there. Open drawers, cupboard doors and closets for better notation. Use the date function on the camera to further indicate ownership on the date shown. Pictures should be filed with the inventory and appraisals of high value items somewhere safe other than in the home. Additional benefits

of doing such a video is to record where family pieces came from. The provenance or story about items pictured, (This mirror belonged to Aunt Minnie who used it in her house in Minnesota at the turn of the century), makes the item more valuable, especially if it is documented. More important it passes on family history for the heirs. **Note:** As I am semi-computer literate and do not own a video camera, I could use our digital camera to film everything and transmit the images directly to our computer. Then I could use a scanner to add all appraisals and sales receipts to the same disc. I can always go back and organize them if and when I need to but at least the information could be stored on a disc with the hard copy and left in a safe place outside our home.

- When listing such things as books, clothes or linens list them generically; i.e. 27 books 12 hardbound, 10 paperback, 5 leather bound unless they are of higher value. For those items, you can list them separately. (Rudyard Kipling, published 1849, etc., 1 satin and lace ball gown, Oscar de la Renta purchased in 1993), etc. Send copies of the inventory to the insurance company and/or some place other than the house for safekeeping. It won't be any help if the only copy burns up with the house.
- Update the inventory when there is a life-changing event such as the death of a spouse, a move, or every five years. Over the years, we have de-accessioned items for one reason or another with gifts to others, selling them, or passing on furniture to our children.

An Inventory is Protection if Home Care or Nursing is Required

It has been my experience that those suffering from dementia syndrome or isolation because of illness will sometimes think a much loved item has been stolen or will give something as a gift to people and then assume it is stolen. The suspicion of theft by home health care workers is devastating, not only to the worker and the patient but to the family as well. Better to store valuable items out of the house with a trusted relative or in a safe deposit box, if appropriate, before workers come or failing that have an inventory. It will help establish the presence of those items if it has been up-dated regularly.

An Elder Law Service Could Help with Planning for the Future

Lawyers who have knowledge of the unique needs of senior citizens and strategies to solve those needs define elder law as their practice. A goal in consulting such a practice is to set up a system helping to maintain control of personal and financial decisions as long as possible and to regulate the expenditures of an estate so there is enough for all one's needs until death. It is also to see that wishes concerning health care are kept in mind when and if one is no longer able to express them. An attorney who is familiar with state requirements can help ascertain that all conditions are met.

Not everyone needs an attorney or financial consultant to plan how to allocate resources in the most effective manner possible, but a partial listing of some of the services they offer gives an idea of issues in our own lives we should be thinking about;

>Retirement planning
>Estate planning
>Preservation of assets
>Disability planning
>Administration and management of trusts and estates
>Health insurance planning, claims and appeals
>Social Security and disability claims and appeals
>Long term care and consideration of retirement downsizing,
>>lifetime care communities and nursing homes

Since time is money for any lawyer, gathering all pertinent information, listing potential concerns and clarifying goals before the appointment may save on fees.

Resource

For a really clear understanding of what an Elder Law attorney can do for you, either send for a copy of their booklet listed below or go to their very informative Website and print out a copy.

Questions and Answers When Looking for an Elder Law Attorney
Send a self-addressed, stamped envelope to:
National Academy of Elder Law Attorneys, NAELA
1604 N. Country Club Road
Tuscon, Arizona 85716-3102—*www.naela.com/naela/questions*

Hundreds of attorneys volunteer their time with AARP legal Services Network to assist with legal questions for the elderly. To volunteer your services:
AARP Connections for Independent Living
Dept. MM,
601 E ST. NW
Washington, DC 20049—202 434-3980—*www.aarp.org/lsn*

Estate Planning, Wills, Trusts and Health Care Decisions

Estate planning is defined as the process of creating a strategy for preserving property during one's lifetime and arranging for its transfer at death while at the same time reducing tax liability.

Retirement and the pension, which financed it, were once relatively simple affairs in years gone by. Taxes were less complicated, medical insurance was straightforward and easy to understand. Now, with the possibility that one could live to age 90 or beyond, it is important to consider whether assets and future needs will come out even. This drives a demand for professional advice to chart a way through the increasingly complex mix of IRA's, Keoghs, pension plans, insurance benefits, annuities, taxes and trusts. In a generation past, it used to make perfect sense to keep savings in low interest bank accounts. Now, there are many more productive places for one's money.

A financial planner can help to evaluate a retirement package and assess how changing careers may affect future financial security or be a guide for reinvesting a lump sum pension payoff for maximum benefit. Although it is difficult to predict the rate of inflation in the years to come, it is something that should be taken into account when planning one's financial future. We are willing to pay our fair share of taxes but we also don't want to tie up what we have if we need it in an emergency. A chronic disabling physical condition should be prepared for even if one is perfectly healthy now. We don't know how long our lives will be or how much help we will be able to give our children and grandchildren, but at least we can think about it ahead of time.

Note: Married or single, anyone dying in testate, (without a will), risks having a government agency decide where the estate will go and who will get what. If there are minor children, the state may appoint guardians and taxes will take a large part of what one would wish to be transferred to them and others.

Financial Planning

This is the process of assessing total assets, liabilities and future income potential, and then using that information to determine the best options for meeting future needs and wants.

Resource

For a booklet which includes information on financial issues;
Planning Your Retirement, Stock # D12322
AARP Fulfillment
EEO 1253
601 E St. N.W.
Washington, DC 20049
AARP also has a website to help you calculate what you will need.—
www.aarp.org/bulletin

Click on "Online retirement calculator"

This is fun and very informative. Designed by the American Savings Education Council, it offers a lot of financial facts and a "Ballpark Estimate" worksheet for all ages.—800 732-0330—*www.choosetosave.org*

Choosing a Financial Planner—
Making Sure it is the Right Choice for You

If one is not skilled in financial management, a way to insure keeping control of one's own affairs is to seek help from professionals who are trained to advise on such matters. It is important that they meet certain criteria. One can find lists of financial planners supplied by local and national organizations. Check each one carefully because the person chosen will be trusted with detailed knowledge of all our resources. There are some dishonest people out there and we don't want them handling our financial affairs.

- Do some homework before the first appointment. Think through what goals are for the future, project what needs could be, and what we wish to leave to charities, children or relatives.
- Ask if the person being considered is a certified financial planner.
- Know ahead of time what your personal requirements and goals are and be able to state them clearly to assist the planner in recommending a plan. A woman must take into account that her earning power might be less than a man's and that there is also a statistical chance she will live longer than her husband.
- Ask how the planner is to be paid. Some represent specific insurance companies or financial institutions so their fees come from commissions on sales. Is there any oversight by that institution? A perfectly good plan may be already in

place so change would benefit the financial planner more than it might the client.
- Always get a written estimate of what services are provided and how much they will cost. It is very difficult for someone to be knowledgeable in every area of concern, therefore ask who the planner will be consulting for the information he or she does not have.
- We should be comfortable and confident with the person we have selected. The ability to explain options in a way we can understand is equally as important as expertise in establishing a good working relationship.

Resource

To understand better what a financial planner can do for you, ask for the free booklet. Expect delivery to be in 4 weeks. Send a self-addressed, stamped envelope.

Facts About Financial Planners, D 14050
AARP Fulfillment
601 E St. NW
Washington, DC 20049

Seeking Peace of Mind for One's Parents Too

In most cases it is difficult for the concerned family to know if an elderly parent has enough resources to live into very old age or if provision has been made for long-term care should it be needed. Taking in and caring for elderly parents or relatives can create a struggle to make ends meet. Even when income appears to be enough for someone to live comfortably and respond to emergencies, the possibility remains that poor investments or uncontrolled spending could deplete what is there.

Financial issues within families are often difficult to discuss and resolve because they go to the heart of some of those freedoms we hold most dear, especially privacy. The ability to make decisions about our own assets, the conviction that we have made the best choices possible with what resources we have is difficult to challenge. If it should happen to me, I can understand why I might resist being questioned about my decisions and the implication that I could not handle my own affairs.

No matter how worrisome a parent's lack of provision for the future, a compromise between a friend or relative offering help and taking over is what we should search for. Concern that inadequate plans to deal with emerging problems as they become increasingly evident drives children to try to find solutions to issues as they surface, which may not coincide with what the person would have chosen for himself.

- If there is a suspicion that plans for the future are outdated or nonexistent, it may be possible to make a case that provisions for tax relief for seniors, trust options, medical insurance plans and investment possibilities are constantly changing, sometimes for the better. It can be pointed out that by taking advantage of these new tools, taxes could be reduced and holdings maximized. If talking about it is difficult put all the information on paper. This helps take emotion out of the discussion and can be seen as less threatening.
- Draw up a list of financial planners and elder law specialists who can be consulted.
- Once the information has been given, back off. It's the hardest lesson to learn. After all, it is their decision to make even though we may feel that they are heading for disaster. It would not hurt to continue to give periodic up-dates on financial issues that could be helpful, (in writing).

Medical and Long Term Health Care Planning

This is a process that helps to assess requirements for the

provision of health care with specific knowledge of federal and state regulations governing public benefit programs such as Social Security, Medicare and Medicaid, and provides for Living Wills, and Durable Health Care Power of Attorney. Health care policy is undergoing constant change responding to market pressures to cut costs but at the same time requiring more knowledge by the consumer in order to get the best care possible.

Some Terms One Should Know

- Health Maintenance Organization, HMO or Managed Care is prepaid health care that has as its goal to provide adequate medical service at a profit by holding down costs. An attempt to cut costs is encouraging plans to focus on prevention and early detection of disease.
- Medicare is a Federal health insurance program for those 65 or older and people with disabilities for which some premiums and co-payments are required. There are two parts, PART A (hospital insurance) and Part B (Medical Insurance). Under certain circumstances, Medicare will pay nursing home costs for a limited time if an individual needs skilled nursing care.

  Note: At this time there is another program being tested in several parts of the country called Medicare + Choice. Ask about it.
- Medicaid is a joint Federal/State program, which pays for medical care for individuals who cannot pay their own medical bills. To qualify for Medicaid, an individual must have limited income and resources and be medically eligible.
- Medigap or Mediplus are private insurance plans that cover the deductibles, co-insurance and other expenses not covered by Medicare.
- Medicare HMO is a managed care program that charges no additional premiums beyond Medicare Part B fees, requires a small co-payment for doctor's fees and provides free prescription drugs, eyeglasses and routine check-ups.

Resource

Medicare Toll Free Hot Line—800 638 6833—Between 8AM and 8PM This is the place to start in order to find a way through the maze of regulations, which shift and change. Call late in the day, as they are less busy then. If one suspects fraud when being billed by a medical service, call the Health and Human Services, Inspector General's Medicare Fraud hot line.—800 447 8477

I have referenced this Website before but it should be done again. This easy to use site, identifies Federal and State assistance programs for the elderly, for which someone may not realize they qualify. This completely confidential website run by the National Council on Aging could dramatically improve quality of life for someone when medical bills are eating away at a limited income.

www.benefitscheckup.org

A Long-Term Health Care Insurance Policy may bring Peace of Mind but Read the Fine Print

Some years ago when this type of policy first became available there was a rush to sign up. Because there were so many complaints of people being victimized, the federal government passed legislation to improve consumer protection but there are still things we need to think through. Consider the odds of ever needing long-term care, your age and health, and the cost. Present and future assets may be enough to cover such costs. We have decided against such a policy in the past because we plan to go into a lifetime care community but it is one of those things we will review again. It is expensive, more so if purchasing a policy over the age of 65 and gets increasingly costly as we get older.

- Make sure the policy reflects government guidelines. If replacing an older policy, which does not embrace the new guidelines, the company cannot place limits on coverage due to preexisting conditions that have appeared since the older policy was purchased.

- Coverage may not be cancelled except for nonpayment of premiums and reinstatement must be guaranteed if payments resume. (This could be important if increasing cognitive abilities cause one to forget payments but requires that a trusted friend be listed on the policy to be notified in that event).
- Long-term care benefits must be paid if two of six tasks of daily living cannot be performed. A person will qualify if cognitive impairment, (dementia, Alzheimer's disease), puts him or her at risk even if 2 of the 6 qualifying tasks have not been met or if prior hospitalization is not needed before then.
- The benefits allowed often do not pay the full cost of home health care or a nursing home. Payment allowed in the basic policy is usually no more than $100 a day for home care and $200 a day for a nursing home. Since a provision of most policies is that one is required to use a certified agency for home care, the allowed amount may cover only a few hours. With nursing home costs rising every year, the shortfall can become very burdensome.

> *An elderly relative paid premiums for a long-term care policy for many years. It was not until several years into her decline due to Alzheimer's disease that my husband discovered her policy specifically excluded Alzheimer's disease and benefits would be $40 per day for one year. Her expenses for custodial care in 1997 were a minimum of $70 dollars daily and increased, as she needed more care. By the end of her life she had required 3 years of full time nursing care.*

- Qualifying for home care benefits can be difficult. Many policies will not provide for a homemaker to assist after a hospital stay for something like a broken hip. To activate the home health care provision, the doctor may have to certify that one is unable to perform two or more of the following activities without help; eating, bathing, dressing, toileting, moving without falling, and getting from bed to chair.
- Payout may be dependent on Medicare approval.

- An inflation clause may make what is affordable now, too expensive later on. If coverage is dropped due to inability to continue paying the premiums, funds already paid may be lost. Ask for an inflation rider of at least 5% a year and benefits, which will last 3 years or more.
- Premiums may be still payable even after admission to a nursing home or if receiving care in the home unless one has a Waiver of Premium in the policy.
- There is usually a lifetime limit to the amount of benefits one can receive therefore one may be responsible for the entire cost of care after a specified number of days or weeks.
- Check the stability and reputation of companies offering such policies. Some have gone bankrupt before benefits could be paid out.
- If a personal support system cannot be counted on for an emergency, there are policies that could be flexible enough to cover a variety of care arrangements such as, respite care, adult day care and home health care, or even payment to friends who might provide that care.
- If deciding to sign up for such a policy, try to do so before age 75 because costs will rise at a lower compound annual rate before then.
- Look for a policy that treats impairments separately rather than requiring a combination of several before paying benefits. If there is one medical necessity, it may not be enough to qualify thus it may be required that one have another problem such as inability to manage daily living tasks or senile dementia.
- Check with a tax consultant to see whether one can deduct some or all premiums along with other itemized medical expenses if they exceed a certain percentage of adjusted gross income.
- Some states offer public/private partnerships where members can qualify for long-term care policies, which can cost as much as 30% less.
- Look for a policy that offers direct cash benefits. Although premiums may be higher, the net cost could be lower because

one could hire private caregivers or pay a family member thus not needing to use an agency for home care.
- Get an increased daily benefit amount if the premiums can be afforded and ask for a higher deductible to cut the cost of the policy. Also consider buying a decreased daily benefit amount if the rest can be covered by one's financial resources.

Resource

Before You Buy—A Guide to Long Term Insurance—Stock #D12893—Allow 4 weeks for delivery
    AARP Fulfillment EEO 164
    1909 K Street, NW
    Washington, DC 20049

This is an excellent guide to deciding whether to buy or not from a non-profit organization.

Long Term Care Planning: A Dollar and Sense Guide
    United Seniors Health Cooperative
    1331 H St. NW Suite 500
    Washington, DC 20005

Planning for Incapacity

This process covers consideration of legal competency, surrogate's decision-making and includes planning for medical needs in the event of one's inability to make those decisions oneself.

Some Terms One Should Know

- A Power of Attorney is a legal document authorizing another person to act as agent or attorney. It is used primarily for financial transactions
- A Special (or Springing) Power of Attorney becomes effective only at a specified time or when there is an occurrence such

as incapacity or if the person designated makes a written declaration that this has occurred.
- Durable Power of Attorney remains legally valid after one's possible subsequent disability and/or incompetence.
- A Health Care Proxy is a document delegating authority for making health care decisions by an individual when an attending physician determines that person is legally and medically incapacitated.
- A Durable Health Care Proxy remains in effect until it is revoked or until it expires upon a specified date.
- A Living Will specifies in advance one's wishes regarding the use of life-prolonging medical care if one should become terminally ill and be unable to communicate.
- Advanced Directives are documents to be used with the living will in which an agent is designated to act on one's behalf if one becomes incapacitated.
- Guardianship is a court-monitored relationship where a guardian has the power and duty to care for property and a person if he or she should become incapacitated.
- Emergency Medical Services Palliative Care/Do Not Resuscitate Order must be signed by the doctor and presented to ambulance personnel if one does not wish to be resuscitated in the case of cardiac or respiratory arrest outside a hospital. (Required in the state of Maryland but may not be in all states)

Resource

Partnership for Caring provides many free resources on its Web site, such as state specific advance directives, living wills etc. and a national hot line for end-or life issues.—800 989-9455

www.partnershipforcaring.org

Why a Living Will?

Executing a living will expresses one's right to refuse treatment that artificially prolongs dying. It can also specify that all measures be taken to keep one alive, no matter what the consequences. Declaration of the "Do not resuscitate" provision in most living wills usually provides for two or more professionals involved in one's care to decide when "heroic" measures will not bring restoration of health to a level where "quality of life" would be acceptable.

A Living Will relieves family members of the responsibility of making such decisions while still honoring the person's wishes. An attorney should be able to explain what is being agreed to when signing a living will and whether requirements have been fulfilled for the state in which one resides.

Note: The U.S. Supreme Court has ruled that competent patients may refuse any and all medical treatment and treatment can be withdrawn from incompetent patients if there is evidence they would have refused the treatment. The Patient Self Determination Act requires health care facilities that participate in Medicare and Medicaid, advise patients of their right to sign advance directives for health care decisions. They also must provide patients a written description of state law and their own internal policies governing patients' rights.

Resource

Tomorrow's Choice—Future Legal, Financial and Health Care Decisions, Stock # D13479
Health Care Powers of Attorney—Stock # D 13895
    AARP Fulfillment EEO136
    1909 K St., NW
    Washington, DC 20049
Planning for Incapacity: A Self-Help Guide
    Legal Counsel for the Elderly/AARP
    PO Box 96474
    Washington, DC 20090—6474
One can download a copy of a State appropriate Living Will and an Advanced Directive or request the documents by telephone.
                      800 989-WILL—*www.choices.org*

Time to Think About the "Right to Die" Issue

Not many of us want to think about our feelings when signing an Advanced Directive or Living Will but there is no better time to address such a decision than when we are healthy and well, not when under the pressure of an emergency situation. Thinking clearly about these issues helps us to assess our attitude about health, quality of life, illness and death. Finances, spiritual values, religious beliefs, and even personal relationships with family and close friends are all things we need to take into consideration when deciding what our wishes are.

Make Sure Everyone is "Singing from the Same Sheet of Music"

Having fulfilled legal requirements to direct the ambulance crew, doctors and the hospital to respect our instructions, we may not have done everything necessary to insure that our wishes are followed. A living will must be executed in the state where we become ill. We must be assured that each doctor and member of the nursing staff treating us in the hospital fully understands how we feel about this most important of decisions. The person holding the Durable Health Care Proxy or Power of Attorney must also be informed of what we have chosen for ourselves. I may not be ready at this point in my life to give up all I know and love therefore it is just as important to leave instructions that I wish everything possible be done to keep me alive if there is any hope of recovery. My definition of an acceptable quality of life may be different from another person's.

The hospital and doctors can decide to ignore such a written request if a family member can make a strong argument to have them do so. We need to see that our family understands and agrees with our decision.

Choosing who will Represent Us

Choosing who will see our estate through the legal process

after we are gone and who will hold our Power of Attorney or Health Care Proxy, says a great deal about how we feel toward those persons if they are so named. It is important to think how one's children would feel on reading who had been chosen to do what, particularly if those decisions have not been shared with them.

> *We had a friend who was putting his affairs in order including writing his will and thinking through who would oversee health care matters if he and his wife were unable to do so. He was concerned about choosing one child over another thus hurting the others. In this case the solution was simple. He had one son who was a successful businessman, (executor of the will), another a doctor, (Durable Health Care Power of Attorney) and another who would be the lead person in the distribution of personal effects and overseeing the sale of the house. As he died before his wife and she was suffering from dementia, his foresight and planning assures her continued care in a way he would have wanted for her.*

Understand what is being asked of the person chosen. Being an advocate or holding another person's Durable Health Care proxy requires an investment in time and a willingness to question every aspect of medical care being given. An executor must meet legal requirements, sometimes go through a huge amount of paperwork and perhaps deal with family arguments over inheritance issues, which is discussed in the last chapter.

It may be more practical to choose someone other than a relative for the task. We may feel that our children do not have the specific skills to do any of the things required or that they live too far away to be able to help. A lawyer friend advised that if it becomes too difficult to share the designations within the family, consider selecting a trusted friend, a lawyer or a bank instead.

- Choose a professional to referee and oversee estate decisions when it is necessary.

- Talk over decisions with each person designated. There should be no surprises when we are not there to explain them and family should feel comfortable with the reasons for making the choices.

Update Documents Periodically

State and Federal tax laws are sometimes superseded by new ones and needs may expand or contract as we go through life changes in our family with births, retirement, grandchildren, and/or deaths. Wills and other legal documents should be reviewed if we move from one state to another or if we have property in more than one jurisdiction. We should evaluate, reevaluate and update documents already executed on a regular basis or whenever there is a change in health, new grandchildren, a divorce or remarriage.

CHAPTER EIGHT

MAINTAINING A CERTAIN STYLE OF LIVING

Retirement no longer means leaving the workforce at a specific time. It also does not mean being of an advanced age as we once assumed it did. In recent years Internet entrepreneurs retired at age 30 and energetic people working well into their 70's and sometimes 80's are still productive and contributing to the economy. Thus we can make no general assumptions about what a person's needs will be for retirement. For some, retirement brings unending opportunities for leisure. For others it may mean another career and for some it will coincide with a time when parents or an elderly relative's activities are being limited by factors that range from chronic illness to an accident or financial reverses. No matter how many times we retire or how well we have prepared ourselves for our own transition from a full time career to retirement, there may be unexpected traumas, challenges readjustments and opportunities.

Middle age and retirement brought us a lot of questions and possibilities to choose from but at the same time we had an aging relative who required increasing care. We found that grandchildren and the time to travel were high on our priority list but fixing a focus for a meaningful use of our time was a little more difficult. Our horizons seemed to be limitless with children no longer in the home and there were many possibilities for taking on projects we had put off for years.

The lines between active middle age and aging, elderly and very old are no longer as clear-cut as they once were. One person I know at 94 has more energy and interests than another one of 70. Clearly good luck and genes play a large part in how well we live our lives but attitude, aptitude, fortitude and gratitude are four personality traits driving some people to be more vital than others and, in effect, ageless. Being positive, keeping one's sense of humor alive, a desire to learn new things, the strength to endure through traumatic events in our lives and our ability to welcome help when it is offered may be as important to our well-being as our genetic make-up. Keep in mind that the law of averages is waiting in the wings to adjust our vision of how we wish to live our lives, thus we may be subject to challenges to our mobility or our ability to see and hear as well as we do now. How successfully we search out options to overcome those challenges indicates the quality of life we can hope to have.

For an example of how some see their own lives, I share with you an email I received from a classmate I haven't heard from in 50 years. It is unedited and unchanged because to do so would be to lose some of the wonderful spontaneity of it.

> *"This old house is silent, her rafters might still ring with echoes of laughter, but I don't hear them. Silence, not complete for I hear the gentle breathing of my sleeping lab. Outside the day is gray and my birds seem to be resting. No distractions. and I am at peace.*
>
> *For a great part of this month I have been blessed with distractions in many delightful forms. Small voices chirping requests and laughing at jokes only the smalls understand. Squeals of delight as ponies perform as their riders request. Watching smalls and their parents clearing my old dead trees from lawn*

and fields. Seeing a two yr. old, man handle a rake four times his height. Watching the smalls mother riding an old race track pony with a smile that lights up our lives.

Having a visit from my beloved sisters children and grandchildren made my life full to overflowing. I painted rooms and recovered a bathroom floor. I shopped and cleaned and tided and got exhausted. the tired disappeared the instant a small face lit up his arms lifted as he ran towards me sure of welcome and loving kisses and hugs.

So for five short days I was given the gifts that only love can supply. My nephew cooked for me, my niece supplied encouragement and love and joy and hours of hard work picking up limbs that she carried great distances to the compost ditch. Then she raked and hauled bushels of dead debris to the same ditch. My great nieces and nephews supplied youthful exuberance that was contagious. Thomas completed a whole pew of us for Easter Sunday. and helped the smalls retrieve barely hidden eggs after church. My daughter Debbie endured five days of pony camp helped by my grandson Andrew and my old act trainer/ now dear friend. so this old soul did not get tempted to lose her cool while attempting to do things best left to younger and fitter hands. All of the above made this visit stress free for this 67 yr old sometimes petulant, gray haired two year old who insists that she can do it all herself. Thank heaven for all these pushy people who do for me what I am unable to admit being unable to do for myself. Oh I love being told not to do while others do it so well. bliss.

My next door neighbor supplied the 83 yr. old end of fifteen from 2 to 83 at our festive food laden table. We ate and laughed and talked in many octaves which complemented each other and made a symphony of joy at Easter lunch.

Encourage Trusting Relationships— Networking Before You Need it

I have embarrassed my children for years by speaking to

strangers in grocery stores, on subways or in airplanes because I have an interest in other people and am often enriched by their stories. If one of the most important factors in staying healthy emotionally as well as physically is to avoid isolation and the resulting loss of social skills then perhaps this delight in people and their stories isn't such a bad habit to have.

Keeping familiar, comfortable relationships alive and thriving or making new ones may take more courage and energy than we want to expend at the time, but not doing so leaves us vulnerable later in life when we need them the most. Many people drift away from social and family ties as they age; old friends may leave the neighborhood to move to a retirement community; a spouse may die or children and their families pursue their own lives and careers far from their original homes. Social isolation can become a serious threat to health and happiness. Having a plan in hand for enriching our lives, helping others and adding to it as we go along could be called "sipping from the fountain of youth" because it keeps us involved, interested and more youthful.

From Experience Comes Wisdom—
From Sharing It Comes Caring

During 32 years of military life when we moved 21 times, I learned the value of making and nurturing friendships for surviving those extended periods when my husband was at sea and for the year he was in Vietnam. Our family, like many in the military, created a support community with new friends, doctors, babysitters and playmates each time we moved. We learned that self-reliance was a valuable commodity but the real rewards came from sharing strengths and encouraging others to do the same. Now that my husband is retired, I found that I have had a need for the same skills in a new community once again.

A relative in her 90's has lost most of her dearest friends and contemporaries so she has encouraged friendships with younger people. Up until a short time ago she had a schedule that would

> *exhaust someone half her age and is mentor/friend to generations of mothers and grandmothers who rely on her unique ability to understand children and bring common sense to the business of raising them. One year she flew to Poland by herself to spend Christmas with her two great-grandchildren and they looked forward to that visit more keenly than they awaited Santa Claus. A key to her success has been her commitment to others, lack of fear of new experiences and the energy to invest in caring for anyone who could use a helping hand. Now, when she needs a little help, all those people she has befriended stand in line to help her.*

A Support System is like having a Savings Account

Whether alone by choice, because of the death of a spouse, divorced, or taken ill, help may be needed sooner than we once had thought possible. Where would we find that help? Thinking through our options as each year passes and being brutally honest with ourselves about what would be available to us practically and financially makes common sense. Even then, the bottom line for people like me is; what can I do now that will assure my independence and a good standard of care should I need it so that my children will not have to worry about providing it?

> *A widow we know fell and broke her pelvis at the age of 83. When asked earlier what she would do if she became incapacitated, she told us that an unmarried cousin would step in to help her if the occasion arose. When the time came to ask for help, the cousin could not leave her own obligations to move in and care for her friend. She therefore was forced to rely on paid caregivers severely straining her limited income.*

Families often do not live close to each other. Adult children may have commitments to their own families and careers therefore counting on them to fill the need when long term illness or incapacity strikes is risky. Relying on having the financial resources to hire caregivers is only one consideration. The most important thing to consider when such a time comes is, who will actually oversee and run the system. When a caregiver doesn't show up for an assigned shift, who will find the replacement to relieve the one going off duty? Overseeing quality of care and watching for signs of abuse take skills that need to be developed. Doing the payroll, Social Security deductions and other paperwork is a daunting prospect requiring a large amount of time.

Census statistics indicate many elderly people are relying on assistance from unpaid non-relatives rather than on hired helpers or paid companions so we know that such arrangements are possible. Examples of this phenomenon are the thousands of volunteers who bring meals to the elderly in their own homes and Hospice volunteers who bring comfort and support to people with terminal illness. But these are often temporary solutions and may have to be amended as conditions warrant. Some communities have established a system of mutual care giving on a day-to-day basis. Churches, clubs, friends, volunteer and fraternal organizations are helping out when families cannot.

Being involved with others of all ages, sharing their struggles, helping them do what they must to stay healthy, or to work through loneliness and depression is an investment in our own future because it teaches us how to avoid the same pitfalls. Keeping relationships alive and well, stepping in for others when an emergency arises, being involved in community activities are all things we can do to keep ourselves well.

Resource

Anyone interested in starting a system using volunteers and volunteer credits for assisting the elderly to remain in their homes can call this agency and inquire how to set it up.

Senior Corps—Tel: 1 800 424-8867—*www.seniorcorps.org*

Designing an Exit Strategy

The entries made in our life's diary are a reflection of our responses to the people we meet, the events we encounter, the challenges we overcome and what we have learned from each other. How we assimilate those experiences and turn them to our advantage shows us that increasing age does not have to mean more infirmities thus decreasing choices.

> *Jodie decided, with some reluctance, to sell her home of many years to her children and move into an apartment in a lifetime care community. A great-grandmother of 80+ years, she drove herself safely and well, baby sat with her grandchildren until they no longer needed it, taught most of them how to drive, started piano lessons at the age of 75, went to foreign affairs lectures, and had a full schedule of daily activities. She had serious health problems in recent years and emerged from each episode a little slowed but with her positive attitude intact. Although she remained in relatively good health and well able to care for herself, she decided to make the move into a Lifetime Care Community before someone told her she needed to be in a safer environment thus assuring that her children would not end up having to care for her.*

We have a number of friends who are beginning to map their future in this way by selling large family houses as their needs for space contract. Moving into smaller homes allows them more freedom to travel and to cut down on increasingly burdensome maintenance. We have seen others who, in middle age, after the children have left home, moved into a multi-story house without giving a thought to the possibility that stairs could someday be a problem in the future. Some are contemplating a time when a lifetime care community or assisted living will be a possibility for their parents but haven't given thought to ever needing such a solution themselves. Those of us who have had the opportunity to see first-hand what happens when living conditions, which were comfortable and familiar for years, became inappropriate in later years because of failing health. We must keep in mind that some lifetime care communities will not accept people as residents who are not able to live independently at the time they apply. If seriously ill or cognitively impaired and thus unable to live independently, joining such a community may not be an option.

When Home is no longer the Castle of our Dreams

We have seen in our own families how a home lived in for years beyond counting begins to outgrow the person who has maintained and cared for it all that time. Making the decision to do something about giving it up is often painful but surprisingly in many cases, people are relieved and can't understand why they didn't do it sooner. It is clear that flexibility is a learned trait and that thinking about it, saying to oneself that someday a move will be necessary helps us to consider alternatives when the time comes.

- *Downsize and/or renovate.* Close off part of the house no longer being used, create an apartment with a separate entrance to rent out or make the present house conform to possible future needs by moving the bedroom downstairs.
- *Sell the present home* and move into something closer to family that is smaller and easier to handle.
- *Home share.* Get together with others who can pool resources and strengths by living in the same house thereby helping each other to maintain independence in a comfortable home setting.
- *ECHO, Elder Cottage Housing Opportunity.* In some communities, special zoning exemptions are allowed for transportable, temporary housing units that are placed on a homeowner's property for the use of elderly relatives and can then be sold or relocated when no longer needed. "Granny flats" are modular apartments that can be used to change a garage into temporary living quarters with the added benefit that they can be outfitted with facilities for the disabled.

Resource

The best information I have found on ECHO is on the AARP Web site.—*www.aarp.org*
        Click on Housing or ECHO.

- *Senior citizen apartment complexes or residential communities.* In response to the growing number of healthy elderly people looking for places to live that are safe and comfortable, there are many such facilities. They usually offer security, transportation, dining facilities, banking, grocery stores, and pharmacies within the complex or nearby.
- *Assisted living.* Also called a personal care or residential care facility, it is for people who need help with activities of daily living, such as cooking and bathing, but don't need skilled nursing services can still maintain a degree of independence in private or semi-private rooms in such a facility.
- *Alzheimer's disease care facilities.* There are an increasing number of facilities that specifically treat and provide housing for people with various forms of dementia including Alzheimer's disease.
- *Continuing or Lifetime Care Communities* These facilities provide a full range of residential options for the elderly. Dining facilities, access to health services, social activities, housekeeping assistance and nursing care ranging from help with daily living necessities in the assisted living section to unlimited long term nursing care are provided.
- *Move in with the children.*

Aging in Place—Renovation

When we built our "dream house", our architect and builder were amused by our insistence on including features that would prolong our ability to stay in the house if our physical needs in the future could limit mobility. When my husband broke his leg a few years later requiring surgery and a long time in a wheelchair and on crutches, that foresight helped him to be more mobile than he might have been. We have an access ramp disguised as a Japanese bridge over a small entry pond.

- All the doorways and kitchen spaces are wide enough to accommodate a wheelchair throughout the house.
- The main living section is on one floor and both the guest room and master bathrooms can be easily adjusted for wheelchair access.
- All outlets and switch plates are within reach of a person in a wheelchair.
- Plumbing fixtures for the handicapped are already in place.
- My vegetable beds in the garden are raised because it is more comfortable to work at that level but it prolongs the time I will be able to garden if I have mobility problems in the future.

Perhaps, instead of moving and starting over, renovation or the upgrade of safety in a present home to adjust to current needs could be a temporary solution to difficulties with living safely and comfortably.

Safety Improvements to Consider

- *Lighting:* Many accidents in the home occur because of inadequate lighting. Use higher wattage or full spectrum light bulbs. Improve lighting on stairs. Place light switches 42 inches from the floor rather than the standard 48. Place illuminated light switches in the bathroom, bedroom, hallways and stairways, nightlights in the bathroom and at the head of the stairs. Put recessed lighting under kitchen cabinets. Experts recommend electrical outlets be 27" from

the floor helping those of us who can't bend over as well as we used to.
- *Stairways:* There are mechanical lifts (chairs, elevators and a moving, mechanical "helping hand") that can be bought or leased for those who find stairs difficult. Ramps and railings will also increase mobility.
- *Around the house:* Slippery scatter rugs, hidden change of level steps, lamp cords strung across walkways and drapery cords that are not secured are an invitation to falls and broken bones. Lever door handles work better than turning knobs for people with limited wrist mobility.
- *In the bathroom:* Install non-slip finish to the bottom of the bathtub and shower. Put grab bars on the tub and reattach towel bars to wall studs so they will hold a person's weight if needed for balance. Using a single-lever mixer faucet with a pressure balanced anti-scald system or adjusting the hot water heater temperature can prevent severe burns. Handicapped toilets higher than standard ones and with armrests if necessary will help people with mobility problems. A shower with a removable sill not only for wheelchair access but also for people who can raise their feet only a few inches off the ground would help. See that there is room in at least one bathroom for a wheelchair to come in far enough to be able to close the door.
- *In the kitchen:* Plan spaces wide enough to accommodate a wheelchair. Rounded kitchen counter tops, shelves on lower levels that slide out and lazy-susan type shelves in corner cabinets are a bonus. Open dishwasher doors are lethal. An elderly friend ended up in the hospital because a painful injury on her leg, caused by striking the corner of her open dishwasher door was reluctant to heal . . . pad the corners. We just bought a new dishwasher that had plastic edges . . . maybe the manufacturer finally understood how dangerous the metal tops were.

Resource

Once again, AARP has well presented booklets on the issue of adapting a house for the needs of the disabled or elderly.

How Well Does Your Home Meet Your Needs?—#D16270
Home Safe Home
Universal Design and Home Modification
The Do-Able Renewable Home—#D12470
The Perfect Fit—#D14823
    AARP Fulfillment
    601 E St. NW
    Washington, DC 20049 — — —Tel: 800 424-3410

This Website has a checklist to assess a house for ease of mobility and safety for an elderly person.
Rebuilding Together—Home Modifications Assessment & Solutions Checklist
                        www.rebuildingtogether.org
The state of Maryland has an office that helps fund and plan accessible renovations using state and federal money for eligible people under its vocational rehab and independent living programs. Look under the title Division of Rehabilitation Services in your own state and try city and county offices as well.

Senior Citizen Apartment Complexes and/or Retirement Communities

The appeal of these alternatives is that they are usually located in an urban setting or near universities where large numbers of people retire and live. Apartment houses where there are a large percentage of people over the age of 60 are sometimes called *Naturally Occurring Retirement Communities, (NORC)*. This type of community allows the elderly to remain in their own apartments by encouraging an old fashioned sharing of concern for others and skills that come from long time friends and acquaintances being together as they age. It helps them manage everything they need to stay independent. Setting up a reliable support program without such a community can be very difficult. The resource below shows how a good program can help to alleviate problems as they appear and make a difference in many lives by the use of resident volunteers earning service credits for their own later use should they need it.

Residents of one large apartment complex have signed up with a program called Volunteer Neighbor Network to give assistance to neighbors who are made to feel confident and comforted that they can remain in place as they live in their own apartments. Services range from helping someone get dressed for special occasions, to picking up groceries or prescriptions, providing transportation to a doctor's appointment and sometimes to spend a few moments passing the time of day with someone every day to see that all is well. The volunteers then gain credits for a time when they themselves may need the same assistance.

Resource

For help in forming such an organization in one's own community write for information. This nonprofit health care cooperative has a bimonthly newsletter and publications on other health related issues. They also offer a health insurance claims service which makes sense of insurance bills in an easy to understand format making bill paying a lot easier. There is a small membership fee and reasonable charges for other services.

>United Seniors Health Cooperative (USHC)
>1331 H St. NW, Suite 500
>Washington, DC 20005—202 783-0588

Home-share or the Nontraditional Home Setting

In this form of living, several people share an apartment or house and contribute to maintenance and upkeep by sharing skills and fees as worked out by the residents themselves. This does not necessarily mean just the elderly could benefit. When rents, sale prices and taxes for housing are high, young people can provide companionship for the elderly and share costs making their housing more affordable also. There are personality issues, financial, liability, insurance considerations and security concerns to be taken into account when choosing the persons to share a home with but the benefits of house sharing far outweigh the loneliness and isolation of living alone for many people.

Assisted Living Facilities

People who need help with some activities of daily living, such as cooking and bathing but don't need skilled nursing services can rent an apartment in an assisted living facility. Meals, bill paying services, transportation to cultural events, companionship and some assistance with personal living needs is provided.

The advantage of such a facility is the ability to remain somewhat independent, with our own belongings around us while getting the personal care we might need to stay active. Although there may be a nurse who can be consulted for health needs, there is usually no skilled nursing facility available.

- We want to look at the contract closely to see what fees and services are to be expected and what the policy is on fee increases.
- We also want to know what the policy is on having to change rooms or when we would have to move out of our apartment into a more intensive nursing or care facility.
- See if the people in the community are compatible and if the physical surroundings are pleasant.

Resource

For help in finding the right facility contact the state or local council on aging and the state's long-term care ombudsman for information.

Try these booklets to help avoid pitfalls in selection of a facility.

Assisted Living: Weighing the Options—Stock Number D17051
Navigating Your Way to a Quality Assisted Living Facility—Stock Number D 17037
    AARP Fulfillment EE01389
    601 E St. N.W.
    Washington, DC 20049
This organization provides a list of profit and non-profit assisted living facilities by state.
    The Assisted Living Federation of America—*www.alfa.org*
    10300 Eaton Pl., Suite 400,
    Fairfax, VA 22030

Continuing or Lifetime Care Communities

People qualifying by age and health can be guaranteed lifelong shelter and access to different levels of health care from independent living in one's own apartment or cottage to assisted living and long term skilled nursing care. One pays an entrance fee and then makes regular monthly maintenance payments that may rise in response to adjustments in operating costs and possible inflation. The lump-sum entrance fee may be entirely refundable, partially refundable, or non-refundable depending on the type of contract. Some organizations are non-profit and others run and owned by for profit corporations.

The benefits of joining such a community range from the ability to be comfortable in one's own apartment or cottage with familiar things, to having someone come in to provide a little help when returning from a hospital stay. When more help is needed with daily living, the next step is to what is called assisted living, usually within the complex. When skilled nursing is needed, the health center or nursing facility provides specialized nursing care. If fear of being isolated in a nursing home someday is one of many people's worst nightmares, this option has the decided benefit, to my mind, of making it easier for friends from the same community to visit at leisure because they live within walking distance. I have seen a devoted husband take dinner frequently with his wife in the health center, bring her down to their apartment for visits and surround her with their friends to keep her spirits up, all without having to get into a car.

There are often many activities available for residents who want them including opportunities to participate in local community cultural events, educational and volunteer activities. Dining facilities, hobby rooms, art and computer classes, bill paying services, limited hour banking facilities, and transportation are only some of the services available to residents.

Some Strategies for Finding the Best Facility: Ask a Lot of Questions

- Is the facility a corporation or not for profit? Is it financially stable?
- Is it affordable? Will the monthly payments rise too fast for a limited budget?
- What are the options for health care should it be needed in the future?
- Do the buildings and living quarters look attractive and welcoming?
- Can I be as independent as I wish?
- Are there interesting activities offered by the facility? Are there too many group activities? Is there an over-regulation of daily life?
- Is it within walking distance of community activities such as the theatre, library or stores and if not, is there transportation?
- Are friends already there and do the residents look as though they would be people we would enjoy?
- Is the climate agreeable? Does it make a difference?
- Are pets allowed? Are there size or number restrictions?
- Are we aware that we will have repeated losses of friends to illnesses and death?

Maybe it's Time to Move

In an ideal world we should reevaluate our living situation at least every five years after retirement or any significant life change such as the death of a spouse, a divorce or a catastrophic illness. Rising housing costs can outdistance fixed income, energy levels may not keep up with the demands of caring for an aging house, and limited mobility can make living on several floors difficult. If our experience with elderly relatives is any example, many people will not be concerned about such issues until they are forced to make a change. I once thought it was just my parent's generation that found it hard to make lifestyle changes but have found people our own age who appear to be destined to follow in their footsteps. An AARP survey found that although older Americans want to stay in their own homes, a large percentage of them do little or no planning for their housing needs in later years. This comes as no surprise to those of us who have tried to solve the complex issue of how to make living conditions responsive to increasing infirmity of older parents or friends.

Selling the House isn't Always Easy

Real estate agents called upon to help people sell a long time residence mention that there are several obstacles that arise in the hope of setting what the seller thinks is an appropriate price.

- Many people have an unrealistic expectation of the value of their property. Often they hear what houses have sold for in the neighborhood and assume that they will be able to get the same thing or more. The problem is that neighborhoods go up and down in popularity and some older houses need serious updating to bring them up to present standards.
- Elderly sellers often are unwilling to face the disruption and discomfort of a cosmetic facelift while they are in the house.

- In some cases there simply isn't enough money to upgrade the house.
- When a quick sale is needed to finance medical or nursing expenses it may not be the prime time to sell a property.
- Even though there is no plan to sell a house now, periodically consult a real estate agent with knowledge of the local real estate market and ask what is needed to a make the house marketable. Think about the possibility of selling the family home in the future and up-date, paint and repair as the need arises rather than having to stretch a limited budget later.

Trying not to Lose Too Much to Taxes

Often a house bought many years ago has increased in value and consequently incurred a larger tax burden. If we have done our homework, we hopefully have found a way to lessen the impact of taxes. An experienced lawyer with knowledge of tax laws can help find ways to minimize the amount given to the government. As we all know, tax rules and requirements change almost with the wind so the following may be out of date by the time this is printed. The safest course is to consult the experts.

- Invest proceeds of the sale into a new home, which, after including all costs of purchase, legal and broker's fees and even possible renovation, is equal to or more than the amount realized from the sale.
- Give a home away through a Charitable Trust. A house can be given to a charitable organization during a lifetime. That organization then sells the house or holds on to it until the donor's death, invests the tax free proceeds and gives a prearranged monthly or yearly fee to the donor or heirs for a fixed period of time. The organization then derives full benefit from the original investment and proceeds. Each state has different laws and conditions for such a trust and

the tax implications are complex but it has been very successful for a friend of mine.
- Sell the house with a lease/option to buy arrangement. Finance the sale of the house for the buyer by leasing it to them until the seller's death at which time the remainder of the pre-arranged purchase price goes to the heirs. This spreads the tax obligation over a longer period of time and gives the seller income for as long as needed. The lessee/purchaser can make any renovations or changes to the property depending on the provisions of the contract.

Moving in With the Children

A survey taken by AARP in 2000 found that around 18% of people 55 and older lived with their children. Many of these people live in "granny flats" or ECHO housing as described in this chapter but most live in the house with their families. It's not a perfect solution for everyone but with work and planning it can succeed.

- Is there a way to have a private apartment with a separate entrance?
- Assess relationships with each member of the family before making the decision to move in. Are respect, love and acceptance words that come to mind when thinking of the people involved? Will it be difficult to fit in with someone else's lifestyle and compromise on big and little issues? Is there room for improvement in the relationship with our child's spouse?
- Sit down with the family before a decision is made. Talk over expectations, household duties, vacation plans, if a pet would be welcomed, privacy issues, social activities, and transportation needs. Finances are always a big issue so the person moving in should establish ahead of time how expenses and the increased workload can be shared. How

will everyone's daily routine be adjusted to fit together as seamlessly as possible?
- Is the house adaptable to someone with possible disabilities such as vision impairment or difficulty walking?
- This is the time to think through options for possible ill health in the future. No one wants to be a "burden" but the possibility exists that as we age, more help could be required for daily living so we have to consider whether the family is willing to take on the extra responsibilities.
- Consider a home-sharing Bill of Rights such as the following;

The Adult Child has the Right To:

- Privacy, respect, independence and control of his or her own life.
- Time to concentrate on spouse and family.
- Support and understanding from the spouse.
- Assistance in making the house run smoothly.

The Parent has the Right To:

- Privacy, respect, independence and control of his or her own life.
- A place to call home no matter how small.
- Feel that he or she is making a contribution to the running of the household.

The adult child does not need to involve the parent in family disputes or expect the parent to assume the role of babysitter unless it has been negotiated beforehand.

The parent does not need to take sides in family disputes or to give advice on how to raise the children.

Resource

There are two books about combined living arrangements;

Where Can Mom Live?—
By Vivian F. Carlin and Ruth Mansberg—Lexington Publishing

This Web site has a lot of good information about housing arrangements for the elderly.

www.aarp.org/lifeanswers

Face the Music—
Moving Day is Just Around the Corner

I write a lot about this subject because I know a fair amount about it but also because from retirement on, the possibility of moving from larger house to smaller or from one location to another is relatively high. If that is the case for you then perhaps it will be worthwhile. I moved many times when my husband was on active duty in the Navy and we made every mistake in the book until we finally got it right. Just about the time I had the whole thing down to a science, he retired and we have lived in the same place for the last ten years so now I share my system with you.

Getting There is Half the Fun

You've lived in the house forever, it seems. Every closet holds treasures that haven't seen the light of day in living memory. There are drawers in chests and tables that won't even open any more and kitchen tools that evoke memories of beautiful dinner parties held decades ago when fancy mixers and 45 bowls to put it all together were used and used again. You always said that you would clean it all out but you just never got around to it and now the house has been sold, settlement date approaches and panic is two steps ahead of the mover.

If you are hiring a mover and have an unlimited budget, you can just pretend that the clutter problem doesn't exist. The packers will pack everything, including your trash, take it to the truck scales, weigh it and send you a bill reflecting the fact that each unnecessary item you had them pack and move will cost you. You will eventually have to deal with it anyway so why not now.

First Things First

Your goal is to make the move trouble free and to save yourself as much effort as possible.

- Place a label on the door of each room with the name of the corresponding room in the new house to which you wish items in that room to go. (You will take all those labels to the new house on moving day before the first item goes in the door so no time is lost telling your movers/helpers where things go.) Make sure you label one room in the old house "trash".
- Visualize your life in the new home and imagine where you are going to place the things that will go into boxes to be transported. That means linens, bric-a-brac, books, art supplies, clothes, etc.
- Take every item you think you will use in each of those labeled rooms to be packed and labeled there. If the movers are packing you or you are moving yourself, this will save a lot of time unpacking when all those boxes will end up where you want them to be. Schlepping boxes all over the house after those strong backs have gone home will slow down your settling in and keep you tired and aching for days.

Now the Hard Part

Remember that room you labeled "Trash"? Divide it into several parts, "Consignment or Thrift shop", "Charitable organization", "Gifts to friends" "Trash". If you have a room near the back door, where things will only pause on their way to their destination, that is the one to use.

- Start cleaning out and organizing your house a room at a

time—right now. My consultant says, "If you haven't worn it, eaten off it or played with it in years, then you do not need it. GET RID OF IT."

- Get boxes from the liquor store. They are a manageable size and you will be able to do your first sorting into them.
- Go through every drawer of every chest, table and credenza then place each item in its appropriately labeled room or section.
- Draw a rough plan of each room in the new house and decide where the furniture is going. You may change your mind several times but it helps you visualize what you will need and what you can pass on or put into storage.
- If you are moving to a place within easy driving distance, transport the comestibles and combustibles to the new place yourself or if not, get rid of them. The movers will decline to move them.

Moving Dynamics

Moving can be a traumatic event. The old saw that a move is equal to a death or divorce doesn't need to be true but it often is. There are several things you can to do to make the outcome more rewarding.

The moving company representative who shows up to estimate your move and tell you what services will be provided and for what cost, is usually the most charming and believable salesman on the moving company's staff. It is his job to convince you that your household treasures will be treated with white glove attention, and that your priceless antiques will be given the care normally reserved for premature infants in a hospital nursery. The business is very competitive and as most salesmen make a percentage of the total cost of your move they will promise you almost anything to get your business. Do not believe this person until and unless you receive assurances in writing that specific measures to protect those high value items will be taken such as crating or packing with cardboard layers, wrapping silver or special photos in acid free paper, etc. You will pay extra for that kind of care but it may well be worth it.

Understand the way van lines companies are set-up. Those huge vans you see along the interstates like Allied, Bekins, Arpin, Mayflower, etc. called carriers, are symbols of nationwide companies and provide basically the same services. Drivers may work for a carrier or be independent contractors who own their own tractors (the thing that pulls the big trailer) but most receive their "jobs" from a carrier. The packers, the agent for the carrier at the point of pickup and at the destination, are the second, third and fourth elements of your move, any one of which, if they are bad apples can ruin your day, or week or year. We have been moved by the best in the business and by the worst but most fall somewhere in between.

The driver usually travels from site to site alone, but is dependent upon the agent who represents the carrier in each place he makes a delivery or pick-up, for the helpers used to assist with loading and unloading the trailer. They may be experienced workers who have steady, well paid jobs or they could have come straight from a hiring hall and never moved a stick of furniture. One of the crew may be a summertime intern who is the agent's nephew, hates the job and knows there is little chance he will be fired for sloppy work. In short, the driver is the boss on the job and carries the responsibility for seeing that there is a minimum of breakage or other damage with your move, but he cannot be everywhere at once. In some companies, a certain percentage of damage claims will be deducted from his pay so it is in his best interest to protect your things. In our 21 moves, we met very few who were not thoroughly professional but when things start going wrong, they often do so because someone took unauthorized shortcuts.

The Packing

Professionals do the packing who are either on contract to the agent or are actual employees and may be paid by the carton. Inquire of the salesman who does the packing. You don't want to be paying for any more boxes than necessary. The estimator is usually good at figuring out how much time it will take to pack your things but be prepared for two people to come rather than the four that you have been promised thus prolonging packing time. Juggling personnel for the multiple jobs an agent is called on to perform, requires that everyone show up for work on a given day and we know that doesn't always happen. Packing is done two or three days before the move out and requires your vigilance in the beginning of the process. Be prepared to have them tell you that they are doing just exactly what the salesman promised and is on your contract, but check and verify as the packing begins to be sure your understanding is the same as the packers. If you don't think so, hold their feet to the fire to get the service expected. If you pack yourself, the company takes no responsibility for damage to the contents.

- Have the packers reserve and label clearly a box for the bed linens including pillows, towels and washcloths, etc. to be used in each member of the family's bedrooms for ease in making the beds that first night.

Local movers operate under a slightly different plan. They rely on reputation and word of mouth for a large part of their business. That means that you would do well to check with the better business bureau to see if there are an unduly large number of complaints against the one you have chosen. Another source of information is your realtor as they often hear a lot about the good movers and the not so good. Again, the driver is usually the boss but not always and you would do well to establish who is the person in charge before anyone comes in the house.

It is the driver/boss who does the inventory. I have rarely found one who inflated the amount of damage recorded on the inventory that protects them from fraudulent claims of moving damage but you need to be aware that such skullduggery does occur. You do want them to be accurate in listing every box, piece of furniture and item being entrusted to their care but it is not a bad idea to scan the inventory as it is being done just to keep everybody honest. It is the inventory that is considered the key reference if you have to place a claim for anything damaged or missing. When you sign it just before all your worldly goods go driving off into the sunset you are agreeing that it is correct in every respect. When you sign it again after your things are delivered, you are agreeing that everything has arrived safely except those things noted on the inventory as damaged or lost during the unloading process. We always signed ours with the statement "Subject to further inspection" because it was often impossible to catch every scratch or broken item during the controlled chaos that is moving day.

Moving Day

- Do not let any member of the crew into your house if you suspect that they are not in proper condition to go to work. Take your complaint to the boss/driver.
- Have chilled soft drinks or jugs of ice water for the people working to access during the day.
- We always ask if we can provide lunch for the crew because, although they often take time for a lunch break, it will be shorter if the food comes to them. Beside which, they appreciate it. A happy moving crew directly relates to a better move! Some people offer a beer to the crew at the end of the job but we do not because, after all, they are driving back to the truck scales and then to the warehouse with all our things in their possession and also it is almost certainly against the rules.
- If you feel that you have a courteous and professional crew, stand back and let them do their job. If you think that things are not going the way you feel they should, speak first to the driver/boss. If you do not get results call the agent. In some cases the move goes well into the time when the office is closed. To solve one such problem, I threatened to tell everyone to leave the house until I received assurances that a problem worker would be removed from the job.
- Before the van arrives at its destination, your new home, have the labels placed on each room with the same names as are on the packed boxes.

- Walk around the house and picture where the furniture is going to be placed. Most movers will allow you to change your mind at least once, but they are not required to.
- When they arrive, ask them to set up a table and chair from the van where you can sit to check off items on the inventory as they are unloaded and from whence you can send things to their proper place. Don't worry if things get a little confused . . . just ask them to wait a moment to let you catch up. It saves time at the end of the day when everyone is tired and you are trying to track down things that didn't get checked off.
- Once they start unloading, just "go with the flow". I liken it to being on a speeding train. It's going too fast to jump off so you might as well sit back and relax.

The Wrap up

Inevitably, some things get broken or scratched or lost. A good crew will help you list those things they and you notice having been damaged, on the inventory. Most claims adjusters know a fraudulent claim when they see it so it's best not to try to pass off damage to a table, which was caused by junior banging his baby cup on it as something found after the move. I won't get into the insurance subject because it is complicated but the only thing you have to know is that the carrier is liable for only a certain amount per pound. If you have high value items, it is best to have supplemental insurance.

If you thought the crew did a great job, email or write the agent involved and send a copy to the carrier. Always list the crew members names because it may make a difference in their job performance reviews. Conversely do the same if you were not happy and be specific in your complaints.

It's Never Too Late to Learn Something New

Keeping up with the world around us implies that we should

learn how to use a computer. If we already have some knowledge of word processing or the Internet, there is still a lot more we could learn. Most people who are younger than I am don't give a thought to using a computer in their daily life for everything from the Internet to paying their bills. I am still concerned about security issues of using credit card numbers and passing on private information on the Internet, but I think they are being addressed. The reality for those of us who years ago thought an electric typewriter was a huge advance is that computers have opened an entirely new world. Our challenge is to move from being apprehensive about learning a new technology to accepting it for what it can do to enlarge and enhance our own experience. There are now programs to help us do tax returns, write wills, do the family genealogy or write an autobiography among many other possibilities.

The Internet is the most easily accessible tool for a layman to research a health problem or for getting the latest information on alternative therapy. News junkies can access daily newspapers from all over the world and the latest stock quotes. Many retirement communities have now added computer classes to their list of activities. It's like learning a new language and skill.

Resource

Microsoft systems has a Web site, which is a wonderful access point for people with disabilities of many kinds limiting their ability to use a computer under normal circumstances.

www.microsoft.com/enable

For Macintosh systems:

www.apple.com/education/k12/disability

Email is a Special Gift for Parents and Grandparents

In this electronic age when communications travel around the world in nanoseconds, fax machines and the computer have changed the way we communicate with each other and do business. Several years ago, when our daughter and son-in-law moved to Eastern Europe, we rationed ourselves to making one phone call a week. The fax machine was useful because the cost of transmission was less than a phone call no matter what the time of day but Email, although not as satisfying as hearing someone's voice, has the advantage of being there when it is wanted. It doesn't have the urgency or disruption of a telephone call and it costs a lot less. The response can be as quick as it takes to sign on to one's Email account to get messages or as leisurely as answering a letter. We now have family in Hong Kong so we will venture into Instant Messaging where communication is, as they say, instant.

The World Wide Web is a valuable research tool for me as I write this book.

Resource

The ultimate in easy to follow instruction booklets which is fun to read as well . . . I recommend it highly.

THE INTERNET FOR DUMMIES A Reference for the Rest of Us!
By John R. Levine, Carol Baroudi, and Margaret Levine Young—
ISBN: 0-7645-0106-2

E-MAIL FOR DUMMIES A Reference for the Rest of Us!
By John R. Levine, Carol Baroudi, Margy Levine Young, and Arnold Reinhold—IDG Books Worldwide—1997
ISBN: 0-7645-0131-3

A Tutor Helped me to get Started

A friend came to our house and explained what I needed to do to access the Internet and then how to use it most effectively. I was surprised that it took a certain amount of tutoring to become fluent in this new language even though I had been using a computer for word processing for many years. Don't let anyone tell you that a computer is a machine of unlimited logic. There is no logic to why it will suddenly freeze and fail to respond to entreaties to move on. I needed someone who could explain what to do, in words I could understand, and who had infinite patience. For one frustrating event, it took our 6-year-old grandchild to tell me how to get things going again. Once I understood the basics, an occasional telephone consult was all that was needed to keep going. We had another phone line installed specifically for computer communications in our home because tying up our one line for long periods of Internet time was unacceptable.

Being a Grandparent. The Best Deal in the World

Parents, children and grandparents bring so many different skills and personalities to the mix that to identify what makes a "good" grandparent is impossible. Grandparenting is an ongoing process shaped as time and events move along. Keeping the "meddle factor" at a low level particularly when it has to do with the way children are being raised is often difficult and requires a sensitive balancing act, at least for me. I have to keep reminding myself that just because our own children turned out well doesn't give me carte blanche to direct someone else how to do their job. We trust and respect our own children's judgment and they, in return, give us the opportunity to participate in their lives as often as distance and timing permit. We can expect certain behavior and standards in our own homes when grandchildren visit but compromising on some things may be necessary to keep the peace. On the other side of the equation, being a grandparent gives me the opportunity to relax the strictest of rules now and then when the grandchildren are with me.

Wisdom that hopefully comes with experience and age has put us in a unique position to be a comfortable "anchor to windward" no matter what the ups and downs of young childhood, adolescence, or adulthood. Our role can be to give unlimited love, support and patience when it is called for.

In theory there are two sets of grandparents. In practice, it doesn't always work out that way for reasons varying from distance, divorce, or illness, to death or estrangement. Finding a compromise between seeing our children's families as much as we would like and respecting the needs of parents for privacy or the other grandparents for equal access can sometimes be complicated.

Resource

For a review of parenting skills and tips on safety ask for a free copy of their booklet call or visit the Consumer Product Safety Commission Website.
A Grandparents Guide for Family Nurturing and Safety—888 878-3256
www.cpsc.gov.
This Web site has everything you ever wanted to know about children's safety.—*www.safekids.org*

When Grandchildren Come to Visit

It may not come as a surprise that we, who have not had toddlers in the house for a couple of decades, have forgotten how much trouble young children can get into. When our grandchildren were first mobile and came to stay with us, I found I was a little rusty on safety issues around the house. In doing research for this book I learned how much I didn't know when raising our own children about keeping them out of danger and how easy it is to make the changes required to create a safer environment. Some parents are more careful than others but the possibility an accident could occur while the children are under our care is enough of a motivator to make the effort. The key for us has been to relax and enjoy their company but to be watchful. Admittedly the following strategies are a little obsessive but they will give an idea of how many things can go wrong if one is unaware.

- Put the number of the local Poison Control Center where it can be easily found in an emergency.

- Ask parents for a list of children's allergies to foods, medicines, animals, etc.
- Devise a fire escape plan for the house then make a game out of training the children what to do in an emergency. Make sure children recognize the sound and know what it means. Tests have proven that they may not react when in deep sleep.
- Even very young children can be taught to call 911 and give their address. Most emergency systems such as 911 have caller ID so even though a younger child might not be clear on what the problem is, personnel could check out where the call is coming from and respond.
- Invest in safety gates for stairways and off-limits areas.
- Avoid toys with small, removable parts that can choke a small child. Check to see that stuffed toy eyes or noses can't come off easily.
- Balloons are a serious hazard when they have popped and are in pieces because they can choke a child when placed in the mouth.
- See that a child wears a properly fitting helmet while riding tricycles, bicycles or those fancy scooters.
- Keep batteries away from children and pets. The acid in them is corrosive and poisonous.

Resource

The Toy Manufacturers of America have a booklet that addresses the issues of product safety, age appropriateness and baby safety. They also have a hotline to report unsafe toys. To receive a free copy;
  The Guide to Toys and Safety—800 851-9955—*www.toy-tma.com*

Safety In the Kitchen

- On the stove, get in the habit of putting pots on the back burners and pot handles out of reach

- Childproof locks for kitchen cabinets are a must for cleaning supplies, medicines, polishes, alcohol, and poisons of any kind. Kitchen stools make what is usually inaccessible much easier to reach for a climbing toddler or young child.
- Electrical cords should be out of sight and safety plugs put in all unused outlets throughout the house.
- The dishwasher should be locked and as an extra precaution never left with sharp knives or soap in the dispenser as they are both deadly.

In the Living Room/Bedroom/Family Room

- Cords for curtains and blinds should be placed well out of reach because of their potential to wrap around a child's neck.
- Stair, balcony and bed railings should be no further apart than 3 inches so a toddler cannot stick his or her head through the slats. Attach strong netting to danger areas.
- Decks, balconies, low windowsills or porches are irresistible climbing and falling hazards. Put window guards on upstairs bedroom windows but if they are part of a fire escape plan have releasable catches.

In the Bathroom

- Turn down the temperature on the hot water heater when young children visit to prevent scalding.
- Bathroom doors and toilet lids should be closed with childproof locks if toddlers are visiting. There are doorknob covers that require the pressure of an adult hand to open the door.
- Hair dryers and other electrical appliances including radios should be put away to avoid the possibility of electrocution if they should fall into bath water.
- Medicines and cleaning supplies should be kept behind locked doors.

Baby Furniture:

- Check older cribs to see that the slats are no more than 2 3/8" apart and that the mattress fits snugly. If more than two fingers can fit between mattress and crib, a baby could suffocate.
- Toy boxes and blanket chests must have safety hinges or be secured so that only an adult can open them. Heavy lids can come down on a child's head or neck and if the chest has no ventilation holes can cause suffocation.

The garage and automobile:

- Trash and garbage can lids should be secured well enough so a toddler cannot climb in and put the lid down. Many are airtight thus creating a real danger of suffocation.
- Place all chemicals, oils, pesticides and fertilizers out of reach.
- Do a safety check on garage door openers. Make sure the safety mechanism is set to reverse or stop if it meets resistance. Test by placing a stiff cardboard box, which could approximate the resistance of a child's body to be sure the door will stop its downward movement.
- Rent, buy or borrow an age appropriate car seat and learn know how to install it properly as the law and common sense require children to be secured even for a short trip. Some insurance companies offer special rebates and discounts when purchasing a child's safety seat.
- Before starting the car, check and double check that every child is safely out of the way. Backing out of a garage or driveway can be a high-risk maneuver with young children darting around therefore move slowly, check and recheck that no one is around. Place a sign on the garage wall in front of the car when children are in residence that reminds the driver to be careful of children.
- When driving with children in the car, keep the distraction level down. I tend to be easily distracted anyway, but I find

that the temptation of sneaking looks at the children can cause dangerous lapses of concentration when on the road.

Miscellaneous:

- Guns should be under lock and key with ammunition stored in a separate locked place whether children are visiting or not.
- Some vitamins and minerals, especially iron compounds can be deadly to children.
- Household plants, particularly those with a milky sap may be poisonous.
- Fire and smoke detectors should be in all the appropriate places and the batteries replaced on a regular basis.

Long Distance Grandparenting

Our grandchildren have lived in Hungary, Poland and now Hong Kong. We try to visit them once a year but we wanted them to keep us in their memory-bank so these ideas could be fun to use.

- Be a pen pal. All children love to receive mail. Email and a postcard for the very young are just as exciting as a letter. But as the children get older, encourage reading skills and active participation by sending a letter with questions and blanks for their answers so that they can mail it back. Send pictures of grandparents, cousins, and friends, pets and places they have visited so that memories of fun times together can be kept alive. Include a self-addressed and stamped envelope for their answers or use a Fax if there is one for a quicker response time, if they live in the USA.
- Start a Book-of-the-Month Club for them. I like this idea. A friend did this and incorporated a tape of her reading one of the books out loud.
- Hearing grandparents' voices, particularly for the very young

and in short segments is a great way to participate in their lives. Have a conversation, sing a song, tell a story about ancestors, or if you are really creative, make a video with other family members to talk about things the children know and recognize.

- Make a book with pictures taken during a vacation visit. Write funny captions for the pictures to remind them of the fun.

Resource

This book comes highly recommended;
The Long Distance Grandmother How to Stay Close to Distant Grandchildren
   By Selma Wasserman—Hartly & Marks 2001—ISBN 0881791881

- Take a vacation with grandchildren. There are several tour groups, which specialize in multi-generation travel arrangements, and some airlines encourage traveling with children by allowing a grandchild to travel free when one is using senior airline coupons.

Resource

This organization suggests tour programs that help grandparents plan trips with itineraries, which will appeal to several generations. Worldwide attractions like glaciers, jungles and mountains, historic sites with castles and ancient cities are offered. They have a wonderful Website

www.grandtrvl.com

This organization will send a free copy of its newsletter and a brochure on an intergenerational summer camp in the Adirondacks. Their Website is loaded with information. Send a legal sized, self addressed and stamped envelope for each.

Foundation for Grandparenting
PO Box 31
Lake Placid, NY 12946

www.grandparenting.org

Being a Substitute Grandparent

When we were the parents of healthy, happy young children it was difficult if not sometimes impossible to find time for shopping, taking a child to the doctor or even grabbing a few moments for recharging our batteries. Now picture what it would be like if one of those children were disabled, handicapped or severely ill. For some families, far from familiar networking systems, isolated from friends, dealing with the stress which comes from juggling all the family needs and trying to give other children a normal existence is to live a life of daily exhaustion and frustration.

The Family Friends Project, sponsored by the National Council on the Aging, matches caring adults with selected families who have severely disabled or ill children. The organization provides trained volunteers who can step in to provide respite care while parents tend to chores like grocery shopping or going to the cleaners. A Family Friend may accompany a parent and child to a medical appointment, read or play with another child in the family or simply be a friend to a child isolated by illness. Specific needs are matched with the personal strengths of each volunteer and special training by health and social workers helps each one to be confident assistants.

I have seen this program in action. I know how much it means to parents and the enormous satisfaction that comes from this type of work for the volunteers.

There is another program called *Foster Grandparent Program* that pairs young people whose parents are unable to provide them with enough love and affection, self-confidence, and the ability to know right from wrong, with the elderly who wish to be mentors.

Resource

The National Council on the Aging, Inc. sponsors this organization. To volunteer or refer a family who needs help call;
Ask for Family Friends or the Foster Grandparent Program—800 424-8867
www.seniorcorps.org

Staying in the Driver's Seat as Long as Possible

Is there a magic age to give up driving? In a word, the answer is, NO. People age at differing rates and driving conditions vary from rural to urban and from city to city. Therefore designating a specific age to stop driving is impossible. Frequency and the distances traveled may lessen as a person's lifestyle changes but knowing when the time has come to lay down the keys for good is such a subjective and difficult decision that some people put it off too long. The freedom to go anywhere, anytime without having to rely on another is viewed by many as a constitutional right. At the same time, failure to recognize that we are no longer able to drive safely can be devastating, if not fatal to others as well as ourselves.

Changes or deficits in vision, reflexes, flexibility or hearing usually occur from the age of 50 on although a person at 80 may be an excellent driver with a good safety record while another at 70 may not. Most people will show signs of measurable loss in these areas around the age of 75. The challenge is to determine for oneself that driving skills have diminished to the danger point. Like so many choices made during a lifetime, this one depends upon knowledge of oneself, courage that comes from making hard decisions and a willingness to find acceptable alternatives to a cherished right.

How Accidents Happen for the Older Driver

- As communities grow, driving conditions change. New traffic

patterns emerge, two-way streets become one way, and there are more signs, more cars on the road and less patient drivers.
- Freeways, beltways, expressways and interstates all require special driving skills, sharp reflexes and constant attentiveness. The mix of high speed, aggressive drivers, "18 wheelers" and now tandem or two trailer trucks makes driving these highways a challenge for anyone but for the elderly driver who is not used to them they can be lethal.
- There are subtle changes in reaction time and reflexes thus slowing problem solving ability. Fender benders, coming too close to the car in front or beside one, repeatedly misjudging distances and hitting the curb are signals we must acknowledge a decrease in driving skills.
- Changes in vision affect driving ability. Cataracts, glaucoma, macular degeneration, failing depth perception and increasing need for sight correction affect day and night vision and may make one dangerously sensitive to glare and insensitive to contrast.
- Reduced flexibility in the neck and shoulders means less vision when we can't turn our heads far enough to see behind and around us.
- Foot problems such as bunions or hip and knee stiffness and pain mean that "pedal speed" decreases, as there is a reluctance to apply pressure to the brakes.
- Borderline mental impairment such as short-term memory loss can cause confusion and erratic behavior. This includes results of the possible side effects of medication and alcohol. Keep in mind that as we age, our body chemistry changes thus magnifying the effect drugs and alcohol have. Momentary lapses happen to anyone but repeatedly forgetting the destination or how to get home push the limits of driving safety.

Driving Experience Doesn't Always Mean Driving Safety

Just because I've been driving for 40 or 50 years doesn't mean my skills are as sharp as they once were. Repeated complaints from a spouse or other close friends about our driving ability could be an important indication that we should take remedial measures or give up driving. There is a good chance they may be right.

Being able to drive safely implies the assumption of responsibility for being physically and mentally competent to do so. Denial is a terrible burden to carry if we cause an accident and someone is hurt. The equation for safe driving changes as we age therefore we must take actions, which bring our skills up-to-date and make us better able to respond to our changing physical condition.

Resource

AAA Local Chapters—"Safe Driving for Mature Operators" Call them for the location of the course and dates. Brochures *Straight Talk for Older Drivers* deal with driving ability, exercises to increase flexibility, and help one recognize problems with vision, medications, and driving while drowsy, car buying and maintenance. Their Web site has an excellent video about senior driving issues.— 800 305-7233

www.aarp.org

8 hour drivers course—Call them for dates and times of the AARP "55 Alive" program—888 227-7669—nearest course.

The Older Driver Assessment and Resource Guide—D14957
AARP Fulfillment EEO1213
601 E St. NW
Washington, DC 20049

www.aaafoundation.org

- Drive frequently. Practice may not make perfect but it does help keep skills sharp.
- Focus on driving. Talking to a passenger or looking at things on the side of the road reduce concentration and can be disastrous. Pull over to the side of the road to use a cell phone.
- Practice defensive driving. Anticipate a problem by watching what cars are doing two or three car lengths ahead.

- "Road rage" is a luxury no one can afford. Being less aggressive and competitive is good for your health and safety as well as those around you.
- Exercise regularly and stay fit as this will help to maintain good overall health and alertness. Pay special attention to neck and shoulder flexibility so that there is full visibility when backing, parking and moving into a stream of traffic.
- Find alternate routes to familiar destinations if the usual ones involve freeways or other areas of heavy traffic. Feeling uncomfortable and fearful of the speed with which everyone else seems to be traveling is a clear sign that we need to find a less traveled route. Driving too slowly and remaining too long in passing lanes on highways can create a lethal hazard to others on the road.
- Be alert to changes in traffic patterns such as new STOP signs or traffic lights.
- Avoid left-hand turns at busy intersections. Statistics show that they cause a lot of elderly drivers problems. Get in the habit of making several right hand turns to get to the same place and to avoid making a left turn.
- Have vision tested paying special attention to peripheral vision and depth perception. Some people experience changes in their ability to change focus from near, to distance and back again. One way to stay alert is to keep eyes moving while checking the road ahead, the rear view mirror and side views as well. Use visual and hearing aids if needed.
- Driving at dawn or dusk or into the sun when it is at a low angle can cause confusion and even temporary blindness. Anyone with cataracts would find such conditions particularly difficult. Do not use tinted glass on side windows or windshield.
- Install an extra large rear view mirror that will improve range of vision and although one should use side mirrors when changing lanes, get in the habit of briefly turning the head to cover blind spots.
- Good visibility means being able to see over the dashboard. The top of the steering wheel should be no higher than the

level of one's shoulder. Get a pillow from an automotive store for the purpose of raising one's line of sight.
- If taking any medication, check with the doctor or pharmacist to become educated about possible effects on driving alertness. Be particularly aware of the interaction between alcohol and prescription or over the counter drugs. Drifting off to sleep while driving is a problem for drivers of all ages but particularly for those taking certain medications. People having problems sleeping at night have a greater likelihood of falling asleep at the wheel. Check with the doctor to see if there is a substitute or another time when drugs can be taken.
- Ask the experts for an evaluation on driving skills and take a course for mature drivers offered by AARP or the American Automobile Association (AAA). The courses are given to people aged 50 or over and teach compensating techniques to overcome problems faced in everyday driving situations. In some states, graduates receive discounts on their auto insurance premiums

If Someone Shouldn't be Driving but Still Is

Some of the most heated discussions I've heard have been between husband and wife or parent and child over a decline in driving ability and safety. The prospect of declining driving skills awakens fears of losing control of one's life and independence. It is also one of the most difficult issues between adult children and their aging parents. There is no easy way to resolve the problem because denial is a potent weapon.

There are usually clues that all is not well.

- Moving violation tickets have been issued for things like driving too slowly, going through red lights or for an increasing number of small fender benders.

- Neighbors or friends call relatives with reports of unsafe driving practices or worse, there is a serious accident.

How can I, as the child of a parent, tell, cajole, or demand that he or she give up driving? How does a spouse tell a loved one that driving with him or her is becoming an exercise in terror? How does a longtime friend explain why driving with someone who can't see well enough is no longer a treat?

Most of us who have been in this position keep our fingers crossed that someday reason will prevail and that either the state will refuse to renew the license or that a particularly frightening experience will force the issue. With testing not required for the elderly in most states, that is an idle hope.

- Confer with the person's doctor and express concerns about his or her ability to continue to drive. If the doctor is willing to advise the person not to drive that may be enough to convince him or her. I have just as often seen someone keep on driving anyway.
- One family added up the costs of maintaining automobile, insurance, fuel, and maintenance showing how much could be saved by selling the car and using local transportation options and that worked.
- Suggest enrollment in driving safety classes offered for mature drivers.
- Taking away the keys may work with some people, but there are not many of us who are willing to deny a person we respect and love the dignity of making their own decision.
- One clever lady gave her elderly parent a book of coupons from a local taxicab company for a birthday present. Another possibility is to draw up a coupon book for our services as driver for a friend to help convince them that they can get around very well without driving themselves.
- As a last resort, if it is your opinion that your parent is risking a serious accident, go to the State DMV and register

a complaint with a request that they retest the person. Ask that your name not be divulged.

Finding Other Ways to get There

- Public transportation, car services and taxis can take the place of a private car and when adding up the costs of maintaining one's own, may be less expensive.
- It's hard to break the habit of being able to go anywhere we want whenever the spirit moves us but learning how to use the above services before they are needed can be considered a training exercise in flexibility.
- In many places, urban and rural, there is a transportation system with home pick-up for the elderly or physically challenged that can be arranged by calling the Eldercare locator, the National Council on Aging or checking the yellow pages for county or city transportation departments.
- Taxicabs can be hired to come on a regular basis one or more days a week so that trips to the doctor, market or friends can be scheduled for those days. Friends and neighbors might be willing to offer rides to the store if they know of the need. One friend I know offered to help a younger friend put all her photographs, which had piled up in boxes and bags, into albums in exchange for rides.

Resource

For help finding transportation of the elderly or physically challenged give the zip code of the person and a referral will be made.
ELDERCARE LOCATOR—800-677-1116

Driving with Disabilities

Thanks to an aggressive campaign to allow people with disabilities access to a fuller life, there are a number of programs and resources available. Being in a wheel chair, or having a disability no longer means that driving is impossible. There are adaptive systems for many needs, some as simple as installing leather or vinyl seat covers for the driver to be better able to slide in or out of the car and as complex as special hand controls. Some automobile manufacturers offer rebates for financing adaptive equipment to help disabled customers meet driving needs in a new car.

Resource

Most domestic automobile makers have some form of financial assistance for people who need adaptive devices for driving a new automobile. General Motors has a comprehensive program for the disabled and those with impaired hearing as well. Other auto dealers should have the information but I found many had no knowledge about any program although the automobile company they represented did have one. Try the dealer first, then call the 800 number for customer service for each make of vehicle and keep digging until you get the answer you want. Reimbursement amounts vary from company to company.

GM Mobility Program for Persons With Disabilities—800 323-9935

SATURN Mobility—800 553-6000, TDD Users: 800 833-6000

They will provide a listing of local driver assessment facilities, local area mobility equipment installers and information on reimbursement if leasing or buying a new vehicle.

Ford Motor Co—800 952 2248

This organization has as its mission "to increase independence for people with disabilities through provision of safe adaptive technologies". Contact them for names of dealers in each state who could modify a vehicle.

National Mobility Equipment Dealers Association

www.nmeda.org

Shake the Dust From Your Traveling Shoes

Traveling, going to new places and meeting new people, revisiting favorite vacation spots, renewing and reviving old friendships, getting away to be away; for those of us who have always enjoyed traveling and even the coming home part, the idea of a new challenge and the fellowship of friends is a lure hard to ignore. If you don't enjoy traveling alone, just can't figure out what to do next, and don't want to miss out on the excitement of new places there are some wonderful travel opportunities combining volunteerism and exotic locations. There are also tours that specialize in interest groups, such as gardeners, dinosaur and fossil enthusiasts, ornithologists, ancient history buffs, wild animal enthusiasts, etc.

Resource

With the advent of the Internet, access to any interest tour is yours but you also can follow the time-honored method of using a travel company or going to the library. For organizations having unusual volunteer opportunities along with unusual and exciting locations;
 Earthwatch—800 776-0188—*www.earthwatch.org*
  info@earthwatch
 Elderhostel Service and Travel—617 426-8056—*www.elderhostel.org*
 Global Volunteers—800 487-1074—*www.globalvolunteers.org*
 Habitat for Humanity Int.—800 422-5913—*www.habitat.org*

Finding Safe and Adequate Medical Care When Far Away from Home

If I am an example of the typical overseas traveler, I trust to blind luck and good health to keep me medically out of trouble. Beyond that, I was never too sure what to do if I had an accident or illness that was serious enough to require medical attention.

- Carry a laminated Emergency Health Care Card. (See appendix) Keep it in a passport so that it will be accessible in an emergency. Be sure that you have included your health insurance coverage with account number, name of company, telephone contacts, etc.

- Be sure there is enough medicine on hand taking into account airport and other travel delays. Check with a pharmacist to learn how medications can be carried safely if experiencing extremes in temperature. Have a letter from a physician listing the names and dosage of each one as some countries are very sensitive about drugs crossing their borders. None of us wants confusion or hassle about our prescription drugs.
- Have vaccinations up-dated, particularly diphtheria and tetanus, and a polio booster for some parts of Africa and Southeast Asia. Check with a doctor or any of the resources below for specific needs for any foreign countries being visited.
- Check with the State Department before leaving and ask for one of their *Consular Information Sheets* that describe a lot of useful information about any country and will also give an idea of the kind of medical care to be found there.
- Checking one's medical insurance policy will clear up any question of whether it covers international care. Inquire about the possibility of a medical evacuation policy for the duration of the trip. Being taken ill in a remote area can be terrifying and it could be very costly to be evacuated to proper medical facilities. There are policies that specifically cover travel emergency situations. Carry a first aid kit appropriate to the area being visited; in other words, bug repellant, antibacterial wound dressings, band-aids, eyewash, etc. Keep a copy of your eyeglass prescription in the kit also.
- Some credit card companies will secure emergency services for their cardholders abroad. Find out what they can and will do in an emergency situation abroad before leaving. Keep in mind that some places will accept only cash thus a credit card may help in getting the cash needed but a low credit limit could be a problem.
- Know how to reach the U.S. Embassy in each country being visited. This may be the best source of information on where to find good English speaking medical care and to facilitate emergency arrangements if they become necessary. Be aware that this is not a free service.

- Carry an emergency passport replacement kit in case yours is lost, stolen or destroyed. Do not carry it in your pocket or purse as that itself may be vulnerable to theft. Photocopy the data page of your passport, have the address and phone number of the consulates and embassies in the countries and cities you are visiting, and two or three recent passport photos.

Resource

I have used these services for a trip to Hungary and found them useful;
    Travel Warnings and Consular Information Sheets
        Department of State Overseas Citizens Service—*www.travel.state.gov/travel_warnings.html*
Names of emergency medical evacuation insurance companies are listed also.

The Centers for Disease Control and Prevention.—*www.cdc.gov*

For information on road conditions in 60 foreign countries;
    Association for Safe International Road Travel—*www.asirt.org*

The International Association for Medical Assistance to Travelers, IAMAT, is a non-profit organization, which advises travelers about health risks, geographical distribution of diseases worldwide, immunization requirements for all countries and makes competent medical care available to travelers by Western trained doctors able to speak in English as well as their native tongue.
        716 754 4883—*www.IAMAT.org*

For travelers with disabilities, this company can set up tours and/or companion travelers to assist them.
www.disabilitytravel.com
For trading houses with someone from another country, this group seems to have the most experience.
www.intervac.com

Jet lag can be Hazardous to Our Enjoyment

There are as many solutions to the downside of traveling to distant areas, as there are people who have experienced them. I repeat some of them here but leave the choice up to the reader.

- Take advantage of massage opportunities now found in many airports before leaving on a long flight.
- Exposure to light at destination waking times before leaving home and at low energy times after you have arrived and are beginning to fade can help. A rule of thumb is 1 hour of daylight for each time zone you have crossed will help set you straight. (We travel to HongKong, which is 13 time zones away!)
- Wear comfortable, non-restrictive clothes for long flights.
- Drink lots of fluids avoiding alcohol and caffeine. Buy a bottle or two of water to take aboard, as beverage service may be difficult to get when desired. Water from airplane dispensers may not be as fresh as one would like.
- Eat foods high in carbohydrates and low in proteins.
- If going to Europe try to find a flight that gets you there at night.
- Exercise as much as possible on the flight and have plenty of exercise at the destination. Life threatening blood clots could form as a result of being inactive for long periods of time.
- If you want to use a substance for light sedation during sleeping times at your destination do so under a doctor's direction.

Turning Disabilities Into Possibilities

Many of us have chronic eye problems that are kept under control by the use of eyeglasses, drops or surgery. Some of us suffer from high frequency hearing loss due to excessive noise during our early years that becomes progressively worse as we age, particularly true of military people and those who have worked around heavy machinery The visual problems are ones we deal with as they occur but there are many who deny that they are unable to hear well because they dread the idea of having to wear a hearing aid. The alternative to dealing with both vision and hearing problems is to become increasingly isolated from friends, to become a danger while driving, and to appear to be suffering from a form of dementia syndrome as confusion brought on by not seeing or hearing properly becomes more acute.

Aids for the Hearing Impaired

- *Telephones:* Some local phone companies and electronic appliance stores have options available for telephones with easier to see dials, and memory phones, one button to push to dial any pre-programmed number. Inserting color-coded indexes on the memory phone—red for fire, green for police, yellow for ambulance, etc., is another aid. For the hearing impaired there is a range of aids; amplified receivers and receivers modified for use with hearing aids, flashing lights to indicate when the phone is ringing, and portable telephone amplifiers for use when away from home. Telecommunication devices for people with hearing and speech defects, (TTY, once called TDD,) transmits a message to a Relay operator who then forwards it. The Relay system is available in many states to assist people with speech and hearing disabilities or the inability to hold a phone.

Resources

This Web site has over 19,000 items for the disabled and includes items for the hearing impaired.

www.abledata.com

To find an audiologist who has been certified qualified to advise on hearing problems check out the American Academy of Audiology's Web site:

www.audiology.org

Look in the State pages of a local phone book for the number of the Relay Operator. In Maryland, the number for assistance is 711.

For more information call:—800 433 2838

Aids for the Visually Impaired

Appliances: Most appliance companies will supply large print instructions for their household appliances. Dealers do not always know of such a service but call the companies direct and ask them for information on how to obtain what is needed

- Computers are easily adapted for people who are having increasing difficulty seeing regular size print as with a click of a "mouse" you can adjust the size of the print to accommodate to the most comfortable reading size for you. Another good reason to become proficient on the computer is the possibility of communicating on the Internet through the use of "chat rooms" making even the most profoundly deaf fully involved in conversations with friends and relatives.

Resource

Lighthouse for the Blind has a licensing agreement with this Web site to offer some articles for the visually impaired.

www.goldviolin.com

This resource is listed earlier in the book but I repeat it here for assistance using a computer.

For a Microsoft system:—*www.microsoft.com/enable*
For the Macintosh:—*www.apple.com/education/k12/disability*

- Newspapers, books and magazines: There are some newspapers and magazines that offer large size print for the visually impaired.

Resource

The New York Times Large Type Weekly—800 631 2580—*www.nytimes.com*
The Reader's Digest—Large Type—*www.readersdigest.com*
Doubleday Large Print Home Library—*www.doubledaylargeprint.com*

This organization has many services for the blind including the possibility of reading the daily newspaper from many cities in the US. Articles of one's interest are read by synthesized voice. The service is free but registration is required.

National Federation of the Blind—888 617 8039—*www.nfb.org*
They also have other resources useful to those with visual problems.

- *Television*: Closed caption service for the hearing impaired has been provided for some time and now there is a Descriptive Video Service, DVS, for those who are blind. Provided free to the viewer, DVS orally describes visual movements, settings, facial expressions, scene changes and body language without interrupting the regular dialogue or sound effects. DVS uses an adaptor called Separate Audio Program (SAP), and is transmitted by many public TV stations around the country and some cable services as well.

Resource

The WGBH Website offers a place where the deaf, hard of hearing, blind and visually impaired can find information and scheduling for public television access. Captioning, and video descriptions are explained.

WGBH
1225 Western Ave.
Boston, MA 02134—617 492-2777, ext 3490
www.wgbh.org
Click on *About WGBH* then on *Services for People with Disabilities*

- *Talking Books:* Finding books on tapes in libraries and bookstores is becoming easier and many people use them while driving long distances. For many years people who qualify have been eligible to use the Talking Books of the National Library Service for the Blind and Physically Handicapped. The Library of Congress will also provide talking books to those who may not be able to hold a book or sit up to read. They have an up-to-date list of books, magazines and newspapers.

Resource

Ask for a catalog of more than 2000 titles and a special, variable speed cassette or disk player with which to play them.

Library of Congress Talking Books—202 707 5100

www.lcweb.loc.gov/nls/

The books are unabridged and selections include fiction and non-fiction, foreign languages and a full range of categories for children and adults. American citizens living overseas can also receive this service.

Making Life Easier Can Be Stylish and Fun

Having just checked out a Website targeting seniors for tools and items for daily living of great design where the words disabled and elderly do not appear, I hasten to recommend it to anyone. If looking for a gift for someone or considering something to solve a problem based on health or mobility needs for oneself, try looking at the Web sites below.

Resource

This organization offers a thoroughly refreshing catalog of good looking items for things from walking sticks to travel, kitchen and gardening items, all for the physically challenged.

To order a catalog:—877 648-8465

www.goldviolin.com

I know so many people who have problems with their feet that I thought this catalog might be helpful.

Footsmart—800 870-7149

www.footsmart.com

Cleaning up our Act

Under the category of things we should do to maintain our style of living but know we won't get around to is dealing with accumulated clutter, which has magically migrated to our closets, cupboards and drawers. While my husband was on active duty, we were forced to clean out our closets 21 times in 34 years as we moved all over the country. It became a habit that I try to follow to this day on an informal basis every year. Recently, while cleaning a closet in my studio, I found several items that had eluded me since we moved into the house ten years ago. Finishing up that room was a breeze because it was more like a treasure hunt. Truth be known, I liked myself a lot more when gazing on clean shelves and seeing the floor in the closets once again. De-cluttering is good for the soul.

Anyone who has been the executor of an estate or emptied a house after a death can appreciate the reasons why organizing pockets of disorder is a good idea. Most of us have things we will never again need or use but we also have family and personal memorabilia documenting our lives that should be preserved and kept together.

- Give yourself permission to work for just an hour to at least get started. Set up a project of a set of drawers, some cupboards or perhaps a closet at least once a week. I find that the time flies and an hour becomes two or three thus it gets done.
- Place things in labeled boxes to throw away or give to charity, seal them tightly and don't be tempted to go through them again. I found that if I took a second look I was doomed and they ended up in the closet again.
- Carry those newly filled boxes directly to the car for transport away from the house. If they go to the basement for disposal later, that's where they will stay.
- Memorabilia, genealogies, professional papers should be gathered in one place and labeled for later organization. Storage of memorabilia requires special conditions to preserve them.

Resource

This book has been well reviewed, if one wants a primer on how to get started on a de-cluttering project.
  Lighten Up! Free Yourself From Clutter
  Harper Perennial 1998—ISBN 0060952652

CHAPTER NINE

Planning the Curtain Call Before the Finale

If we have learned anything from our friendship with elderly relatives, as I have documented in previous chapters, it is that overcoming challenges to quality of life issues gives each us the privilege of making our own decisions and the grace to welcome assistance when it is needed. For what is perhaps one of the most precious gifts we can give our families, there is nothing more generous than to plan how we wish to leave this earthly life. One of my reasons for writing this book was to help people understand that preparing for the consequences of one's own death is an act of perfect reason and a gift to the survivors of unexpected thoughtfulness. After all, what could be more inevitable? As I have mentioned before, when my mother died, we were faced with learning a lot of things in a hurry, none of which we had been prepared for. Hospice was there for us during the last month of her life and we knew we could count on that organization to give us the support we needed for the end of life and grieving process. What we were unprepared for was the need to document her life and to notify the proper people who had been a part of it. Who knows how many we missed? We neglected to send a death notice to the city newspapers where she grew up and another city where she spent 35 years of her life.

Resource

Partnership for Caring has a national hot line for end-of-life concerns—800 989-9455

www.partnershipforcaring.org

When writing the first chapters of this book, I showed them to a friend, a retired Navy admiral, who gave me several pieces of advice. I have used many of them but the most valuable gift was a paper he had written called, *Bereavement Assistance Notes Planning for Present Peace of Mind*. It was written with the military retired person in mind but there were some important plans of action included that would help anyone, some of which you will find below. When a loved one dies, no matter whether there has been a long illness leading up to that event or if it is sudden, whether it is in a health facility or in the home, there are certain formalities that must be observed. In his words; "This compendium is aimed at assisting surviving family members at the time of a loved one's death. Personal accounts affirm that this is a time when grief hinders logical and prompt action. There tends to be a paralysis of thinking, which is exacerbated by frustration in locating personal papers." I can personally attest to that.

Resource

This Website has a very good checklist of things for the surviving spouse of a military member to do at the time of death.

MOAA "Survivor Checklist: Help for Loved Ones"

www.moaa.org

This is also a useful list for survivors.
AARP "Final Details: A Guide for Survivors When Death Occurs"—D14168
AARP Fulfillment
1909 K ST NW
Washington, DC 20049—Allow six weeks for delivery

Putting Everything in One Place

Appendix A at the back of this book is a guide for collecting the information needed for someone to put our affairs in order after we die. If you have not already done something like this before, do it now. The next step is to tell a trusted friend, lawyer or relative where these papers have been placed to make them readily available when needed. Retired military persons and their spouses are due certain benefits that might not be apparent to others. A listing of the information needed to claim them, how to find out more about each benefit and whether we want to take advantage of any of them could save a lot of effort for the survivors.

Where There's a Will, There Should Be a Way

In Chapter Seven I wrote of planning ahead and gave definitions of various legal instruments for doing that. An up-to-date, legal will tells how we wish our property to be distributed and also names the executors and person we wish to administer any trusts we have set up

A Will is Not a Document for "Getting Even"

Aside from its obvious purpose, think of a will as an opportunity for peacemaking, if it is needed. It can be a document for encouraging a sympathetic and understanding relationship of heirs with each other and for allowing them to celebrate their relationship with the person writing it. Putting ourselves in the position of beneficiaries reading the will makes it easier to consider how they would perceive the regard we hold for them. Hopefully if there has been estrangement, it would have been dealt with before death. Prolonging the pain by slighting some and rewarding others after we are gone can be considered a luxury in self-indulgence.

One child may be doing better financially than the others thus tempting us to leave more to the less well off. Experts suggest that, once again, each child should be treated the same thus avoiding the perception that we wish to reward the unsuccessful while slighting the one who has "made it". If loans have been made to one child, and not to another, our estate could forgive the amount of the loans while the other could have his portion increased by the same amount. Favoritism for one child over another can cause pain and family disruption long after our deaths.

Why Perpetuate the Myth of the Ugly Stepmother/Father?

Second marriages can create major problems for inheritance especially where there are large amounts of money involved and children of two marriages. Assuming that we have kept our assets in our own name, each can leave their own things to their own children. If that is not the case and money will be needed to take care of the surviving spouse then a *QTIP trust* can be set up allowing the income from the trust to take care of that person's financial requirements as long as needed. Under this arrangement, the principle eventually will go to the children of the deceased spouse. We may think it is no one's business but our own what we plan to do with our assets when we are gone but many of us have seen how step parenting can be full of misperceptions and misunderstandings.

Clearing the air before a new marriage with a marital contract is one way to make things clear but if the heirs do not know what our decisions are and how they fit into those plans, then putting the facts down on paper, which they will not see until the parent's deaths, will not ease the concerns of that first family that it has been taken into consideration. Once again, actions speak louder than words but words and an understanding of how much these issues mean to each family are what make for greater peace. The dynamics between children of a first marriage and the parent's spouse in a second one are difficult enough.

Of course there is the possibility that our heirs may have their minds only on our worldly goods, but the bottom line, it seems to me, is that they do not want to be replaced in a parent's life by a new partner. They may not fully understand the concept of our ability to hold them as close and dear as ever, while at the same time opening our hearts to others. It is our responsibility to see that we make that clear to them. I have found from other adult children's bitter experience that it is important to spell out what family items or personal mementos of the parents should go to children of the previous marriage. Having to establish the right to share family mementos after death of that parent is deeply painful for both families.

Things as simple as picture albums and fishing poles, or embroideries done by a parent can be treasures to that person's children and should be treated as such by stepparents. Where there is a second family, children who might hold some of those same items just as dear, would feel just as entitled to them. Solve as many of those problems long before needed by circumstances and allot them by letter to each participant in the family. One couple I know solved this problem shortly after their marriage by asking the children from previous marriages to come into the home and pick out the family things they treasured most before the two households were combined. Those items, which the couple did not feel the need to retain, were distributed. A list was kept of the others and a letter of instruction was written so that minds were eased that those things, which had a family history, would stay with family.

Thinking of the Grandchildren

Consider also whether grandchildren should benefit from our estate. If one parent, our child, dies after inheriting proceeds from us, the possibility exists that the estate could go to the surviving spouse who then might remarry and spread the estate among new and additional family members. If this is not what is wanted, a Totten Trust, a generation-skipping trust, stipulates that certain specified assets would go directly to grandchildren at a time we think is appropriate. The person named as trustee would be entitled to use the income and some principle for the benefit of the grandchildren. This does not require a written trust document and costs nothing to set up. One should get advice from an expert in this type of trust to understand the requirements and limitations but at this writing, the assets would go tax-free to the beneficiaries.

Resource

This Website has clear concise explanations of trusts with the proviso that it is only for education.
    Baptist Bible College and Seminary

                                                    www.bbc.edu

---

The Last Step may be the Most Important

A will may not be necessary because of the way an estate has been set up or if there are no assets to be transferred, but those cases are rare. Whatever system we use, we should talk to our children about how we intend to leave things so that there will be no misunderstandings or false hopes. Losing a parent can be very painful for the adult child. The will should not add to the grief.

Remembering Friends with Personal Gifts

Sharing things we own after death, which have a relationship to people we have known and loved, is a generous thing to do. Giving them to the person while we are still on this earth is a pleasure and gives one the opportunity to know they are safely where they belong. This is also an opportunity to make inanimate objects take on a value far greater than their appraised amount. Some of the furniture, family portraits, jewelry and even bric-a-brac have a history of their own that should be passed on with the object itself. A *provenance*, meaning source, tells the story of the item, where it has been, who made or bought it and where. This is not a time when accuracy is important but it helps to have receipts or reference to an inventory. Some people write information in a letter of instruction, others write it out and paste the facts securely on the back of the object. A letter of instruction is a less formal document than a will but also another indicator of our wishes to be followed by the executors.

Remembering the kindness of those who would not normally be left a large gift by allocating a meaningful memento gives our passing more meaning. Though heirs are not legally required to make good on bequests if they exceed assets, a clause could be included excusing them from making such a gift if it cannot be found or if there isn't enough to cover a cash gift. If you have executed such a document, be sure to up-date it if you make some other disposition before your death.

As with any important papers, find a safe repository for them preferably not in the house and tell a trusted lawyer, friend or heir where they can be found.

Resource

This book clearly sets out problems that could come up when writing one's will. They are presented in easy to read format and treated with a light hand. The book is not a substitute for a lawyer but does make one aware of things we may need to consider.

Beyond the Grave: The Right Way and the Wrong Way of Leaving Money to Your Children (and Others)
Jeffrey L. Condon & Gerald M. Condon—Harper Collins Publishing—
ISBN 0-88730-703-5

Being an Executor. It's Not Always an Honor

A friend calls to say that he is working on his will and would like to name me an executor of his estate. My first thought would be that I am touched anyone would think of me for such a trusted position. In the cold light of day however, I remember my husband's duties when he served as executor of his aunt's estate and my own when I shared duties with my brother and sister as an executor of my mother's will. I realize that for a complicated estate with varied assets, it can be a time consuming job for a year or more.

- Before accepting the commission I would ask the person if he has made it clear to the family or a trusted friend where a copy of his will is kept. Does someone other than this person know where information on financial and business figures are, and how to access everything needed for closing out his estate? I would also want to know if the heirs are aware that I am being named as executor and are comfortable with it. If hesitant to address these issues, I would seriously consider declining.
- Be prepared to do a balancing act. One needs to become current on tax laws and legal responsibilities, hire a lawyer, be able to make business decisions in a field in which we may have little or no experience, and at the same time show tact and wisdom in balancing the wishes and opinions of the heirs.
- Dealing with officialdom brings lots of surprises. One must get more certified death certificates than could be thought necessary to have on hand for closing out accounts and establishing that contracts must be terminated. It is truly stupefying to find how many one must have. In some cases the funeral director will provide the copies.
- A lawyer is required for estate settlement in some states and a good idea in any case no matter how skilled we are in financial dealings. Errors could cost a lot more if something

is incorrect than it would have to consult with a lawyer in the first place. Be sure the lawyer is well versed in tax matters and laws in the state where the estate is probated. My siblings and I ran up huge bills because we didn't understand what had to be done by a lawyer and what we could do. Ask right up front before the clock starts clicking. Keep in mind that every phone call to the lawyer is billed to the estate including cheery conversations about the weather or how the children are.

- All assets and liabilities of the deceased must be inventoried. (It is to make the job easier for the executors that you have gathered all your important papers in one place) A date-of-death balance must be listed for all savings, checking, IRA, etc. accounts and a valuation on stock and bond portfolios, personal belongings, furniture, jewelry, etc., and real estate holdings.
- Protecting the estate from loss during the probate process is the executor's responsibility and one has a fiduciary and legal responsibility to do so to the best of his ability. The heirs have a special interest in decisions that are made with the possible unpleasant result that they could hold you liable for any sizable loss to the estate.
- Have an accountant review income tax returns for the previous three years then ask the IRS to conduct an expedited audit of the estate tax return and issue a closing letter to the executor that the return is valid before the estate assets are distributed.
- Distributing proceeds to beneficiaries takes place after taxes have been paid and all creditors attended to. Since the executor can be held personally responsible if all the assets have been distributed and other claimants come forward, careful attention to detail, and legal assistance is usually required. Getting all those papers and bills pulled together sometimes takes a huge amount of time particularly if the deceased did not organize them ahead of time. Some states

have rules set up to safeguard the executor so find out about them.
- Sometimes one gets a fee for services. We have never taken any but it is perfectly acceptable to receive a legally set fee when the estate is complicated and requires a large amount of time to settle.

Resource

Some of the information from the section above came from USAA and a booklet they distribute when asked.
Duties of an Executor—The USAA Educational Foundation—
1 800 845-0291
A book they suggest for the first time executor;
How to Administer an Estate: A Step-By-Step guide for Families and Friends
By Stephen G. Christianson—Career Press—2001—ISBN 1564145239

The Funeral—Having it Your Way

It's a fact of life that as we get older, we go to a lot of funerals. I have been to some as sumptuous as the Triumphal March from Aida and others as simple as dropping a wildflower into a grave on a windswept hillside. All of this has led me to think about how I want to ceremonially leave this earth. I have always felt that I would not like to stand up and choke back emotions in front of friends and loved ones while saying the things I feel very deeply about someone close to me being gone. So I would not want anyone to have to do that for me. Perhaps a booklet to be handed out at a memorial service might be the right note with a few quotes from friends and family. I do want to have the benefit of clergy and I want lots of flowers, especially wild flowers and lots of beautiful greens with berries and textures. I love music and there are some particularly beautiful lines from scripture that would be comforting, with my favorite prayer of St. Francis. I have tried to convince friends that it is not depressing to think like this. I feel as though I am planning an event or a family reunion. It's creative and satisfying to imagine how things can be eased for my family by taking the details off their minds when there will be so much else for them to think about.

Resource

The most comprehensive book I have found on all aspects of death, rituals surrounding it and grieving. Very insightful;
Remembering Well: Rituals for Celebrating Life and Mourning Death
By The Rev. Sarah York—Jossey-Bass—2000—ISBN 0-787955078

That's the Easy Part. Now for the Details

- Is my obituary written?
- Have I made a list of newspapers I would like it to go to?
- Have I picked a funeral director? Have I pre-paid for the funeral or have I kept aside money for that purpose in a savings account?
- Do I want to be cremated or be placed in a casket? Will it be an open or closed service? Do I know what casket or box I want and have I paid for it? Do I have the contract and the receipt? Where?
- Do I want a religious service and if so, where? Do I want pallbearers? Do I know who I want to conduct the service?
- Do I have a gravesite bought and paid for? Where is it? Do I have the contract and receipt? Has a gravestone been ordered and paid for? Do I want planting on the site? If so, is it permitted and what kind do I want? We will be buried beside the Severn River at the Naval Academy. Perhaps we'll have a bench as a marker so people can sit and enjoy the view, which includes the house we built and lived in for

many happy years. (Haven't gotten that far in planning the details with my husband, yet.)
- Having answered these questions, have I told anyone else what my decisions are?

The Obituary—
How I Would Like to Be Remembered

When my mother died, we were so caught up in our daughter's wedding, which occurred three weeks later, that there were several important omissions in our efforts to do what was expected of the survivors when a loved one dies. We omitted important facts of her life and didn't send it to all the newspapers we should have. There is nothing morbid about writing one's own obituary. In fact, there could be no better time to write it than when the thought of death is only a philosophical exercise. Not only will it be insurance that our life's accomplishments will be truly and accurately represented but it could be an opportunity for us to review them ourselves.

Look at death notices in the newspaper for the form of an obituary then fill in the spaces. Go ahead and list everything if you want to, (such as "Served as den mother for Girl Scout Troop 316 in 1958 in Beverly Hills", or "Graduated from American International School in Singapore in 1955"). If it is important to you then you have a perfect right to put it down. Our family might find the things we list of some interest and they can decide what they want to include in the obituary when the time comes. The newspaper will edit it further anyway so put it all in.

Whom to Notify?

Who do I want to know that I have died? Who, of my friends, would be a comfort to my family and would want to know about a memorial or funeral service? Who do I care most about and who needs to know that I cared enough about them to have them on the list? If my family went through my address book for clues, they would be hard pressed to know my good friends. They know the obvious ones but there are people I hold very dear who I never see and who aren't in my address book. Again, it's like putting together a Christmas card list. Some friends I rarely hear from and others never fail to tell us they care. Those are the people I don't want to forget so it is my job to put together a list and leave it where it can be found with the other decisions I have made about what to do in the event of my death.

What about a Prepaid Funeral?

It is possible to plan ahead for one's own funeral and prepay for it at the same time by signing a contract with a funeral director of choice. In my research, almost every reference, not written by funeral directors themselves, advises against it for the reasons listed below but it is something to look into even knowing the pitfalls.

- The contract may be very complex with hidden clauses and requirements therefore leaving the heirs to struggle with additional charges at a highly emotional time.
- The company contracted with could be out of business by the time death takes place.
- The family may be told that a casket already paid for is out of stock thus an effort could be made to talk heirs into one that is more expensive.
- If death occurs in another state the contract may not be refundable and if it is it may not include interest.

I won't be there to see that my heirs get what I paid for so the contract should be where it can be readily found with other papers before funeral arrangements are made. A safe deposit box is not a great option, and although the will could give some information on my wishes, it probably won't have the documentation one would need.

Suggestions were made by those who have been through the process that it may make better sense to place an amount we feel would be needed in a money market account or look into something called a Totten Trust that will pay a beneficiary at the time of death to fund funeral expenses and is tax free. Although we may have left funds to pay for the funeral in our will, there needs to be money that can be drawn on shortly after death rather than having to wait for the will to go through the probate process. Find out costs of the kind of funeral wanted, caskets or boxes in which to place the remains, the fee for other services such as preparing the body for cremation and add some more for contingencies. Once again, the last part of the process is to tell our children what we have done and where all the information is.

Live On and On as an Organ Donor

As an organ donor, we have a unique opportunity to bestow the gift of life or sight to someone who desperately needs it. Those who have made that decision for a dying loved one during a time of profound sadness, and those who choose to make that decision for themselves in order to provide life for a complete stranger, truly understand the meaning of being selfless.

There is also a program for living kidney donors. Since a human can manage well on one kidney, and because the benefits of a live donated kidney help in the overall success of a transplant, this is a very much-appreciated gift. The main requirements to qualify are good health, a matching blood type and to be psychologically comfortable with being a donor.

Our families should know and agree with our decision to be organ donors if we decide to do so. At the same time we, and they should know about procedures and obligations. The survivors should never be charged for any services by the hospital or surgeons once death has occurred. That includes services performed in order to evaluate the viability of any organs or tissues for donation and keeping organs alive although the patient is certified brain dead. Hospitals have been known to make mistakes in their final bills so they should be checked carefully to be sure there are no inappropriate charges. Before making any designation, consultation with a local or national donor organization will answer any questions and set up the proper procedure.

Resource

For the most comprehensive Website on the subject I have found, this site gives a listing of the organization to contact in ones own state.

www.organdonor.gov

An organization, which can assist donor families, is the following:
Association of Organ Procurement Organizations
1250 24th St. NW, Suite 280
Washington, D.C. 20037

Grieving is a Survival Skill

There are many life experiences where we suffer loss. I can reflect back on a period when at a very young age, my canary, which I loved dearly, flew away because someone left the cage door open. I grieved for a long time and the fact that I still remember that incident with a certain pang is evidence that loss is felt keenly even by the very young. I grieved each time I left my grandmother and grandfather at the end of summer visits. While I was growing up, I suffered from real pain when a series of beloved dogs died of old age. After I married, each time we moved from some place where we had lived and loved wonderful friends, I learned how to grieve again and again. When my mother died, I was so caught up in relief that she was no longer suffering, in planning for our daughter's wedding and the official duties of my husband's job that my sense of loss and the resultant grieving didn't really surface until months afterwards. But when it did finally hit me, I suspect I went through all the classic stages written in books about such matters. If the end product of grieving is the lessening of pain and the continued enjoyment of flashes of memory about the person being grieved for, then it can be said that I have successfully walked that path, let myself through the gate and moved on to other challenges.

Suffering from terminal illness is a continual grieving process complicated by the fact that even the best of doctors cannot predict precisely what course an illness will take with each individual. The power of the spirit, of a person's will to fight and live and the different effect of medications on each body changes the equation daily. I know that spirit exists and have felt warmed and comforted by it when I should be the one doing the comforting. For the family of an Alzheimer's patient, grieving is a lengthy process made more difficult by the presence of the living body, the shell of a person once known.

I have been told that acceptance of death makes us more sensitive to the beauty of life, of moments of warmth and friendship, of color and form and the music of awareness. What could be a better way to think of loved ones who have died than to see with crystal clarity the gifts of life they gave to others?

Resource

This book has many insights on one person's view of his own dying. It changed my thoughts on death, not only my own but beloved friends who have died.
Signs of Life—A Memoir of Dying and Discovering
By Tim Brookes—Times Book/Random House 1997—ISBN 0-8129-2468-1
The Hospice Foundation provides comprehensive and compassionate assistance with grieving to millions of people. Look in your local telephone directory for the Hospice office near you or go their Website.—*www.hospicefoundation.org*

Although I have listed AARP for many resources, once again they provide another excellent resource.

www.aarp.org/griefandloss/

Helping Others Help us Grieve

I cannot begin to tell anyone else how to deal with loss. Grieving is an essay we write ourselves. But I can tell you, from experience, that well-meaning friends deserve to be told how we wish them to help us. When a friend's mother died, I found that the hardest issue was to know when I was doing something helpful and when I was being a pest. A friend told me that finding the words to describe what is needed is a difficult thing to do. People are anxious to help and some shy away from seeing a person going through the pain of grieving and in some cases do too much. She told me that we must be clear about how we can best be helped. If we don't want to see anyone, make it clear that we wish to have the time to find our way alone before seeing people and assure them that we will call when ready. She suggests that when having the urge to talk, find a "spur of the moment friend" and don't hesitate to call him or her. If people keep asking you out or dropping in when you would rather not see anyone, tell them you are warmed by their concern and love but that you are not ready for socializing . . . just tell them. She said the most comforting words she heard were, "I'm so sorry."

Leaving a Legacy

Having become a grandmother, I am sensitive to my place in our grandchildren's life. I am aware of the link, the connection in the chain of life from which they came and a part of the even longer chain of those who will follow us.

I read somewhere about the anguish of a young woman who had been away with the Peace Corps when her grandmother died. She was unable to return before relatives came in to clean out the house for its sale. They had saved virtually nothing that she felt would help her remember this vital and loving woman and the happy times she had spent with her. She didn't want the furniture or the silverware or any of those things. What she wanted most were the photographs and some of the books she remembered reading during happy summer visits in her childhood. Now every trace of this special person except the memories has been wiped away.

That story made me think of the obvious; things like legacies and wills and photo albums but also of other ways to keep alive one's place in family history. It brought back memories of happy times and special people, of sadness and trauma, of world events and local happenings, of friendships strong and relationships gone. I began to think of the adventures I had shared with my husband during his naval career, the tough times when he was gone for long periods, the rewards of community projects completed, and the beautiful places visited over 32 years in the military together.

I have gone through many family albums handed down over the years with pictures of people long gone and no one left who can identify any of them. I feel a responsibility to those who follow me to identify the hundreds of photos from my own life in boxes in the closet. I want to know where my ancestors came from and what they did with their lives but the piles of memorabilia I have are disorganized and deteriorating so I will have to move fast.

Writing Memoirs Validates a Lifetime

My life has been full and I have been privileged to participate in many interesting events but an autobiography, a factual chronology of my entire life, would bore me as much as it would future generations who might someday find it nestled in a box of musty, yellowed remnants of photos and papers. The recording of memories, and combining them with photographs is much more appealing to me. I want my children to know that I did interesting things in my life and I want to remind myself that I made a difference in the lives of others. Never mind that I am not a well-known author, the skills are not as important as the putting down of important events as well as the little ones, the impressions I had of the people around me and what I remember of history being made during my life.

An article from the AARP Bulletin of November 1997 had some hints on how to begin putting our recollections down on paper.

Refer to picture albums, home movies, or childhood memories to get started.

- Think about family stories passed on over the years. Remember personal accomplishments, missed opportunities, and even embarrassments.
- Give the story a beginning, a middle and an end.
- When a memory comes, write down as much as can be remembered then file it away to be fitted into the whole piece later.
- Create a scene the reader can "see, hear and even smell". Include details like who, what, where and when.
- Describe what people say, their personalities, attitudes and if it makes sense, their appearance.
- Be willing to be honest about mistakes, blunders and making some wrong decisions. Our descendants want to know that we were real people and it allows them to put their own momentary lapses in proper perspective.
- Don't hesitate to laugh at yourself. A sense of humor makes a much more enjoyable experience for the reader.
- I have to get over the feeling that my life experiences are any less interesting than someone else's. It's up to the reader to make that call.

Resource

This sounds like a good source for help in getting started.
> Turning Memories into Memoirs: A Handbook for Writing Life Stories
> By Denis Ledoux—Soliel Press, 1993—ISBN 0961937327

This site has a number of questions to get you started. I found the format particularly good for using photographs and doing captions by asking questions to jog the memory.

www.capturingmemories.com

Bringing the Family Out of the Closet

Over the years we have received copies of family genealogies from relatives we hardly knew. I put them away and vowed someday to do something with them. I have found letters written by my great, great grandmother when she was being courted by my great grandfather, and a copy of a land grant in Hot Springs, Arkansas signed by William Garfield as President. The question is . . . what do I do now? Classes are being offered in community colleges, senior centers and libraries on how to do a genealogy, write a family history, and conduct interviews of one's relatives. The Internet gives us the opportunity to access records all over the world. How do I get started?

Decide What Approach to Take

- A genealogy lists the names of our ancestors.
- A pedigree chart is the way to keep track of the order and relationships of those ancestors.
- A family history tells their stories.
- An oral history is the verbal recounting of personal stories and history
- Personal papers and memorabilia are the evidence of one's history.
- An obituary is a biographical notice of death.

Doing a family history was my choice. The hardest part was deciding where to draw the line. In the boxes that are piled up near my desk, there are wedding certificates, birth notices, letters to business associates, love letters, ordinary day to day business letters, and a pedigree that purports to be from 1542. They are from both sides of my family. Am I going to do a genealogy later or a pedigree chart? What do I do with the papers that document these lives? It seems that one decision suggests many more questions.

I must gather all the material I can lay my hands on. I have asked family members to search their attics and closets for any material on family and send photocopies if they want to keep possession of the items themselves. I have asked them to label everything they can.

- Recording research carefully and accurately is a given, but deciding if the information I have is genuine is a problem. Passed down genealogies are only as accurate as the persons recording the information chose to make them. Double-checking with two or three sources helps solve the problem of incorrect entries and official records such as birth and marriage certificates are helpful. Start with what are known facts.
- Family history passed down through the generations may be more legend than truth. Don't get hung up on trying to prove something that can't be documented. If it is part of the family lore then it should be recorded as such but facts should be recorded with footnotes and bibliographies.
- Expand the search by using the Internet to include distant relatives not known before and use message boards to communicate with people of the same name from all over the world. One can access libraries and genealogical societies all over the world.

Resource

If you enjoy doing research online the Church of Jesus Christ Latter-Day Saints offers an incredible wealth of genealogical records where one can search for information on ancestors.—*www.FamilySearch.org*
Another useful online source:

www.familytreemagazine.com

Since doing genealogies and family history has become popular in the last few years, there are many "How to" books out there;

The Genealogist's Companion & Sourcebook A Beyond-the-Basics, Hands-on Guide to Unpuzzling your Past.

By Emily Croom—Betterway Publications—1994—ISBN 1-55870-331-4
The simplest guide I have found for getting started is a book written for children to help them do a genealogy.

Roots for Kids, A Genealogy Guide for Young People
By Susan Provost Beller—Genealogical Publishing Co 1997—
ISBN 0 8063 15253

Using the computer and going Online to do a genealogy is useful but novices need a little help.
GENEALOGY ONLINE, Researching Your Roots
By Elizabeth Powell Crowe—The McGraw Hill Books, Inc.—1996—ISBN 0-07-014754-X
National Archives and Records Administration has a very helpful site giving information on doing genealogical research, how to get started and how to access their records.

www.nara.gov.

Finding a Place for Professional Papers and Pictures

In going through relative's closets and attics, we have found many professional papers and old photographs. Trying to figure out what to do with them is difficult. There is a good chance that they have been resting in the same boxes where they were placed when the owner retired from the office or assignment or job. They were saved for a reason and perhaps bits and pieces might be more important than a first glance would show. The immediate reaction is to feel that no one could possibly want all that paper, but the fact is that they may hold the missing key to a complete picture of some historical event. All it costs is a phone call to the historical association of the area in which our ancestor lived, the company for which he worked, the university with which he was associated or the military service in which he served. Don't throw away history . . . let the experts make the decision whether the papers are worth saving but at least go through them and eliminate duplications, label pictures and attach memorabilia. Then offer them to an organization or some family member to whom they would be important.

Veteran's History Project at the Library of Congress

There is a project to preserve the accounts of men and women involved in World War I, World War II, the Korean, Vietnam and Persian Gulf Wars. There will be a "national archive of experiences and documents for future generations." AARP is a major sponsor of this program and is working with the American Folk Life Center of the Library of Congress. It occurs to me that in one of the boxes of memorabilia I have to go through is an account of my Cousin Olive Leslie who was an ambulance driver during World War 1 in France. I wonder if they would be interested. The original account of her experiences is in a military library collection but perhaps they could use a copy. We have boxes and boxes and scrapbooks of photos from my husbands 42 years of Navy life. They have not seen the light of day for at least 10 years but neither of us has the heart to throw them away. Maybe this would be a place to start to go through them and send them where they could be valued.

Resource

To contribute memories, recollections, photos, video recordings, letters, personal accounts or anything else that would relate personal experiences contact:

Veteran's History Project
Library of Congress/American Folk life Center
101 Independence Ave. SE
Washington, DC 20540-4615—888 371-5848
www.loc.gov/folklife/vets

Storing, Preserving and Protecting our Treasures

All of the memorabilia, papers and photographs from both sides of my family sit in the room where I write this book. The only thing to be said for the attention taken to their care is that the temperature remains fairly constant. The cardboard boxes they are in almost surely hasten deterioration of the papers contained in them, as do the plastic bags in which photographs were placed to keep them together. Before they came into my custody, there was little done to keep them from light, water or mildew damage, all of which are devastating to their longtime preservation. If there is any thought of handing them down to family, I will have to do better.

- The first step is to see what I have.
- Since there are several families, I want to separate everything into separate archival boxes.
- I must order proper boxes and photograph albums in which to store things made of proper archival materials.
- Being completely ignorant of how best to preserve what I have, the next step is to educate myself through the best resources I can find.
- See that humidity and temperature in the area mementos are stored is constant. Low 70 degrees and approximately 50 % humidity are just about perfect.
- Avoid exposure to light.
- I have found some good reference books and will work now to save what I have.

Resource

Since the largest part of my cache of memorabilia is paper and photographs, this book caught my eye.
An Ounce of Preservation: A Guide to the Care of Papers and Photographs
By Craig A. Tuttle—Rainbow Books Inc.—1995—1-56825-021-5
This is a more complete guide for storing all kinds of memento including dolls, wedding dresses, and porcelain.
Caring for Your Family Treasures: Heritage Preservation
By Jane S. Long and Richard W. Long—Harry N. Abrams, Inc 2000—ISBN 0-8109-2909-0

Clearing Out a Family Home Can be an Emotional Roller Coaster

Selling a home filled with memories of happy family gatherings; of childhood experiences and associations with a beloved parent can be a time consuming and saddening experience. We have cleaned out and organized the sale of two large family homes and helped another family member prepare her mother's house for sale. Struggling with the death of someone we love, especially a parent, does not make the job any easier.

In one case, a relative had saved every piece of mail she had received in the last 5 or 10 years; every circular, every receipt from the store, every piece of scrap paper, and every piece of wrapping paper and ribbon from years of Christmas presents. One room was so crammed with full trash bags that it was difficult to open the door to go in. It took over a year of steady work to go through this three-story house with all it's closets, attic and basement, checking each bag and each scrap of paper to be sure that nothing of value or importance was thrown away. As she had suffered for many years with Alzheimer's disease, she had hidden money all over the house necessitating the opening of boxes, looking in books and purses as well. She had lived in the house for 70 years and there was clothing and memorabilia from her earliest years in the house to be gone through and distributed. It was a sometimes exhilarating job as a treasure or a photo marking some event in her interesting life was unearthed but it was also exhausting driving home the hazard of letting things accumulate.

Don't Let the Enormity of the Project Overwhelm you

- Assess the amount of work to be done. Think of it in terms of manageable allotments of time; a closet a day, a chest of drawers, another, and it gets done.
- If the job is to be done after death, and after allocation of the items in the house has been decided, be sure family

members and heirs agree on a plan of action for doing the work.

1. Clear out one room or section of a room for each beneficiary, and mark that section or room with a color sign coded with each individual beneficiary's color tag. When the division has been decided, each person's items could then be placed in the room designated for pick up. Have another place for bric-a-brac of uncertain value. (At the end of the process, friends can be given a choice of items in which the family is not interested)
2. Mark the items to go to each person with their assigned color tag and take them to their designated location in the house.
3. If decisions have been made on which items are to be sold and given away, have the organizations taking them do so as soon as possible. Do an inventory of items going to charitable organizations for later tax deductions and have the driver sign it with the date when they are picked up.
4. If more than one person is to go through papers set up a place in one room with a long table, if possible and have clearly labeled boxes where items can be placed for further sorting. Since deciding what is trash is a judgment call, do not throw anything questionable away until it has been double-checked.

- Rent a dumpster for the trash. It saves a lot of wear and tear to be able to collect the discarded items in one place over a period of time rather than on scheduled trash days.
- If clearing the house comes when someone is moving to a smaller home assess how much help is needed and wanted. Leaving a house in which a lifetime of memories resides is an emotional experience for all concerned. If a deadline is not looming, and we want to help as much as we can, we

have to take clues from the person doing the moving. Sometimes all that's needed is to take notes to be referred to later but the hardest thing is to hold back from doing the things *we* think need doing. There will be a time when our services will be valuable but most times we have to wait to be asked. There are times when waiting is not practical. We had the experience of clearing a house for an elderly friend when a settlement date was fast approaching and the person selling the house was physically and emotionally unable to do what had to be done. It was a very difficult task for all concerned and had unpleasant repercussions for years to come.

Strategies for Sharing the Memories and the Valuables

I can think of no single event after a parent's death that can cause more anger and discord than the division of valuables in the family home. Normally rational and warm relationships can become strained when members of the family get down to the serious business of deciding what they *have* to have and what they think they *ought* to have.

In speaking with a lifelong bachelor at dinner one evening, he mentioned that he was having trouble deciding who should get some of the things from his considerable collection of old books, antiques and memorabilia. He worried that his nephews had shown no interest in family things or for the antiques he had so lovingly collected over the years.

This is not the first time that I have heard this complaint. My mother years ago, as she was beginning to think about these issues, made pronouncements about what each of her children would want. I will admit that at the time she was right about many of them. What she did not take into account was that the association with her and our childhood was more important than any *thing* itself. She made assumptions based on what she saw in our houses and the way we lived our lives then but by the time she died 30 years later, we had all moved on to another phase in our lives and our memories of her dictated our wants. It was only because we were willing to discard her lists and sit down together to work it out amicably that the tangible evidence of her lifetime and its relationship to our lives went to those to whom it meant the most.

> *Many years before my mother died, she had all the furniture, silver, and paintings appraised for insurance purposes. At that time she circulated a list of all the items, but without their valuations, to each of us and we were asked to pick what we would like to have in the future. We received a copy of the allocation list after she made the determination of what she wanted to give each of us. At the time of her death 30 years later, we consulted our lists and found that some of the things we thought we wanted then were not what we wanted when she died. By mutual agreement we decided to scrap the lists for the time being and try another approach as described under "Two Ways to do the Selection" below. The obvious benefits of this approach is that we had a list to go back to if there were problems, each of us felt that no one was getting a better deal than anyone else because we all ended up with some of the things we really wanted and we learned something about each other as we went along. We never lost sight of the wish to respect the memory of a very special lady and to celebrate our relationship as siblings.*

As our lives change, I find that there are belongings in our house that mean a lot to each of our children. It rarely has to do with monetary value. It has everything to do with how they feel about their childhood, their parents and the homes they have known as we moved from place to place during our time with the Navy. Although storage may be a problem in their smaller houses or their lifestyle may not call for some of the things we want to give them now, we are trying to "de-clutter" our lives and wish to save them the taxes they would have to pay at our deaths. Although we wish to be in control of distributing our own things, I have seen the hurt that comes from an elderly relative giving away treasured family things to others outside the family who might not understand the significance of the items. Again, it is the link with family, with those who came before that is important to most people and we will try to honor our children's wish to be a part of it.

Two Ways to do the Selection

- We went through the house, listing the items we wanted in each room in order of our individual preference and then came back for a conference. When two or more picked the same thing, we went back to look at the item in question and assigned a "degree of want" category;

    1. I want it because it is an important memento of my relationship with my mother or father.
    2. I want it because I have always loved it.
    3. I want it because it will look great in my house.

Another conference narrowed the contested items down even further and "horse trading" finished off the rest. The last step was to see that everyone got the same amount in monetary value although we did not do this because we were satisfied with how things worked out.

Another way to do it

- Each room containing items to be distributed is assigned a number, as are the beneficiaries. Drawing numbers decides the room in which one will have first choice and the order of choosing. Some people specify in their wills the persons having first, second and third choice throughout with other family and favored friends coming in later. The strategy used above will still work using this method.

There are many more ways to create a fair system. The ones here appealed to me because they took out of the equation monetary value and helped to avoid the illusion of one person getting more than another. Another thing to keep in mind is that even though a beneficiary may state no interest in the selection, the children or grandchildren should be consulted to see if they would like to be remembered in some way.

Keep it Simple

It is usually a good idea to have the direct beneficiaries participate without spouses, children or advisors attending the actual division. We consulted with our spouses before the selection but specifically avoided having an outside expert come in and tell us the value of each of the items. Although an inventory and valuation was required for tax purposes we found that it was not very reliable in terms of resale value.

Give Some Things Away Now

As long as limits to the exemption of gift tax are observed, heirs and beneficiaries could enjoy the use of the pieces we want them to have while we are living.

Preserve the Memories

Do a video of the entire house and garden or surroundings before the break-up of the house begins while there is still a sense of the person who has lived there and before the house becomes a shell. Do a running monologue, tell stories, remember events, record for all time the life that made the house a home, and give our families a memory they will treasure. Have a family gathering and do the video together to make it even richer. If you haven't the expertise for such a project, hire someone to do it for you.

Lessons Learned When Clearing a House

This is the time when we discover that saving is not necessarily a virtue. Ane of us who have had the job of clearing a house for an estate settlement, understand the need for keeping ahead of the clutter long before the need to empty a home becomes clear.

> *I remember going to an elderly cousin's house after her death, to register the items I wished to receive, as a beneficiary of her will. My maiden cousin had lived in a turn of the century, four-story house for at least 80 years. Every surface was covered with figurines, metal dishes, porcelain flowers, pincushions, lamps with lace shades . . . it was like a museum but I could see it was going to be a nightmare to clean out. In the attic were individual rooms for storage, each one filled to the ceiling. In one was a treasure trove of hats, all in their individual boxes; there must have been 100 hats she had saved from her earliest days. In another room were huge storage drawers filled with kitchen utensils. I stopped counting eggbeaters after 81 and potato ricers after 35. She was an early recycler; there were drawers and drawers with rubber bands, and smoothed out, used aluminum foil.*

When there are no living beneficiaries, lawyers will often contract with a business to come in and clear out a house, saving things of obvious value to be sold but throwing the rest into the trash. I can't bear to think that the bits and pieces of my life and those who have gone before me would be indiscriminately tossed out. I need to winnow out the extra clutter, to simplify our life and give the children the pleasure of using things they have an association with now, not after we have gone. Nothing could be more of a motivation to me to give away those things now than to think of them going to an auctioneer or into a dumpster.

And so the Finale is a Beginning

In my late 60's, in good health, energetic and filled with gratitude to be all those things, I finish this book with a sadness that comes from actually finishing it and having to let it go. It has been my constant companion for many years as I kept adding material and learned more about each subject.

There are things I advise the reader to do throughout this book; to plan ahead, to organize a lifetime of paperwork and memories, to learn new things and open oneself to life's opportunities. It is now time for me to pursue all those possibilities and to "practice what I preach". It has been a consuming passion to share what I can with my friends to keep them from repeating the innocence and lack of preparedness with which some people of the generation preceding us have moved into the last years of their lives. Most of us have a lot to learn about the process of aging and if this book challenges us to gain the knowledge it takes to welcome each new stage in life, I will have succeeded beyond my wildest dreams.

APPENDIX A

PERSONAL AND BUSINESS INFORMATION

Date completed . . . .

Name . . . .   Date Birth . . . .
Address . . . .
. . . .   Nationality . . . .
Tel   . . . .
                                    Naturalization . . . . . .

Social Security Number . . . .

Parents
Name . . . .   Date and place of birth, death
Name . . . .   Date and place of birth, death

Marriage status   Spouse . . . .
Widowed . . Divorced . Legally separated . .
                             Place of birth . . . .
Dates . . . .   Date of birth . . . .
                             Nationality . . . .
                             Social Security # . . . .
Children
Name . . . . Date of birth . . . . Address . . . .
Name . . . . Date of birth . . . . Address . . . .

Military Service . . . . . .   Dates of service . . . . .
Rate or Rank . . . .   Service # . . . .
VA claim # . . . .

Family records are kept:
Birth, marriage, divorce, discharge papers, naturalization, etc.

Lawyers
Business . . . .   Personal . . . .
. . . .
. . . .

My/Our will is located . . . .
Executors . . . .   Address . . . .
. . . .
Tel . . . .
. . . .   Address . . . .
. . . .
Tel . . . .

Power of Attorney . . . .   Address . . . .

Terms:
. . . .
Tel . . . .
Durable Health Care . . . .   Address . . . .
Terms:
. . . .
Tel . . . .
My living will is: . . . .

Employment . . . .   Dates . . . .
. . . .   Dates . . . .
. . . .   Dates . . . .
Membership in private clubs, organizations, etc.
. . . .   Account # . . . .
. . . .
. . . .

Funeral and Burial wishes;
    Instructions;
        Headstone, cemetery, religious service,
        Pallbearers

Obituary
List of persons to notify with addresses and telephone numbers

FINANCIAL INFORMATION:

Bank . . . .   Acct. # . . . .
    . . . .
    . . . .

Where cancelled checks and statements are kept . . . .
List IRA, Checking, Savings, Money Market, CD's etc.)

Safe Deposit . . . . . .   Acct. # . . . .
    Key is kept . . . .
Financial (Cont.)

Savings Bonds, denomination and type, date of maturity
Stocks, bonds and securities, (attach statement or list where they are kept)
Real estate ownership, personal, business, and rental contracts
Location, loans, insurance, acct. #s, mortgages due dates for payments

Credit cards, charge accounts names and #'s
Life Insurance, company type, policy #, value
Health insurance, company, type, policy #
Homeowner's and liability insurance, type, policy #

Annuities, (govt. & commercial), type and name
Pension, employment benefits

Military, retirement pay, other benefits
    Finance center location, tel.
    VA payments, benefits, claim #
    Regional office, tel.#

Social Security payments
    Acct. #, Regional office address and tel.

A copy of your most recent income tax return or where to find it.
List and location of valuable jewelry, furniture, silver, etc.

APPENDIX B

Emergency Health Care Information

Name . . . .
Address . . . .
. . . . Telephone Number . . . .

Person to be notified in case of emergency

Name . . . .
Address . . . .
. . . . Telephone Number . . . .

Social Security Number . . . .

Military ID number . . . . Status . . . .
Insurance Policies
Name . . . . Number . . . .
Name . . . . Number . . . .
Medical Health Information
Blood type . . . .
Drug allergies or sensitivities . . . .
Illness or conditions being treated
. . . . Doctor . . . . . . Tel . . . .
. . . . Doctor . . . . . . Tel . . . .
Medications presently being taken
. . . .
. . . .

Primary care doctor . . . . Tel . . . .
Dietary restrictions, allergies . . . .
Legal and personal instructions

Copy of living will enclosed in packet
Copy of EMS Palliative/Do Not Rescuscitate Order (If required)
Person holding Durable Health Care Power of Attorney, Proxy
Name . . . .   Tel . . . .
Address . . . .
. . . .

Designation if you are an organ donor

APPENDIX C

EMERGENCY HEALTH CARE CARD

Your name, Home address and telephone number
Nationality and Passport number and place of issue
Conditions for which you are presently being treated
Your doctor's name, address and telephone number
Blood type, allergies, drug sensitivities, medications being taken
Insurance policy, company, type and policy number

SOURCES

This listing does not include sources already named and referenced in the text. I think it is important to note that a lot of useful information can be found in newspapers and magazines. I have to add a caveat. Just because information is in the public sector it is not necessarily accurate or complete, but is only as good as the writer's understanding and knowledge of the subject. Obviously any conclusions drawn (whether it be in a book, magazine or newspaper) come with the writer's bias. Finally, although some of the sources were printed years ago, the information they provide is often as pertinent today as it was then.

Chapter One

Wall Street Journal, Dec 31, 1997—"Who's Afraid of Aging? Usually Not the Elderly—They Know Better" By Clare Ansberry

Parade Magazine, April 26, 1998—"How (And How Not) To Age Well" By Gail Sheehy

Parade Magazine, April 20, 1997—"Can We Grow Young?" By Ronald Klatz and Carol Kahn

Washington Post Magazine, June 1, 1997—"Longevity"

Parade Magazine, May 23, 1999—"Live Now, Grow Old Later" By Dr. Isadore Rosenfeld

Chapter Two

New York Times, March 21, 1999—"No Longer an Age, but an Expanding State of Mind"

Modern Maturity, Sept-Oct 1999—"The Facts of Life" By Ken Budd, "Intimacy 101"

By Barbara Mathias-Riegel, "From Lib to Libido" By Susan Crain Bakos
Parade Magazine, May 17, 1992—"When It's Time For a Change" By Ed McMahon
Retired Officer, March 1999,—"Planning for Your Retirement" By John Miller

Chapter Three

Washington Post/Health, Jan 23, 2001—"Adding a Little Iron to Your Life" By Therese Droste
Prevention Magazine, Feb 2000—"The Best of Nutrition Online"
Washington Post/Health, Nov 3, 1998—"Portion Distortion" By Lawrence Lindner
Washington Post/Health,—"How the Body Changes with Age"
Cooking Light Magazine,—Explaining a Low-fat Cookie's Label"
The Capital, Oct 13, 2002—"Hidden Dangers" By Kim Severson
The Washington Post/Health, Jan 23, 2001—"Adding a Little Iron to Your Life" By Therese Droste
Cooking Light, May 1997—"Going through the motions"
AARP Consumer Guide #1—"How To Be Drug Smart"
The Washington Post/Health, Sept 21,1999—"Supplements that Don't Add Up" By Lawrence Lindner
Eating Well, Oct 1997—"To Your Health" By Peter Jaret
Cooking Light, May 1997—"Sweet Dreams are Made of This" By Richard Laliberte

Chapter Four

Washington Post, May, 1995—"The Healthy Personality" By Don Oldenburg
Wall Street Journal, Oct 10, 2002—"Going Online to Make Life-and-Death Decisions" By Laura Landro
Wall Street Journal, Nov 12, 2001—"The Best Way to Get Reliable Health Information" By Laura Landro

Wall Street Journal, Oct 19, 1998—"Do Your Homework: How to learn about your doctor-before you pick one" By Robert Langreth

Modern Maturity, Sept-Oct, 1995—"The Dream Team" By Dr. Joyce Brothers

Cooking Light, Nov 2001—"Be Your Own Medical Advocate" By Melissa Ewey Johnson

Vital Signs, Anne Arundel Medical Center—"Women and Heart Disease"

Retired Officer, Feb 1999—"When the Brain Attack—" By Marilyn Pribus

The New York Times, Aug 10, 1997—"Now, Prescribing Just What the Patient Ordered" By Sheryl Goldberg

AARP Bulletin, Feb 2003,—"Help Yourself to Seconds" By Susan Jacoby

AARP, May and June, 2003—"I'm afraid I have bad news" By Elizabeth Austin

Washington Post/Health, March 26, 1996—"Surviving Your Hospital Stay" By Consumer Reports on Health

Life Magazine—"See Me, Feel Me, Touch Me, Heal Me" By George Howe Colt

Modern Maturity, May/June 2001—"Shock Treatment" By Pat Palmer

Chapter Five

Washington Post/Health, Oct 13, 1998—"How to Avoid Crime by Home Health Workers" By Thomas M. Cassidy

The Guide to Retirement Living—"Home Health Care Services"

The Retired Officer Magazine, Sept 1995

AARP Bulletin, Dec 2001—"Care managers emerge as new force in helping" By Linda Greider

Modern Maturity, Jan 1993—"Home Alone" By Frances Leonard

Washington Post/Health, June 5, 1990—"Rules for Checking Out Care in Nursing Homes"

Chapter Six

New York Times, July 5, 2000—"Less Aggressive Treatment Urged in Severe Alzheimer's Denise Grady
Washington Post, April 1, 2002—"Alzheimer's Patients Get Medicare Break" By Helen Dewar
National Institute on Aging, NIH Publication no. 93-3433—"Multi-Infarct Dementia"
The Wall Street Journal, Personal Journal, July 17, 2003—"When Caring for Aging Relatives Stirs Emotions you Wish you Didn't Have."

Chapter Seven

The Guide to Retirement Living—"What is Elder Law?"
USAA Magazine, Jan-Feb 98
Town & Country Magazine, August 1998—"Estate Planning Without Tears" By Denise M. T Topoliniki
The Retired Officer Magazine, April 1998—"Financial Forum" By Lt. Col John Miller.
Retired Officer, Dec 1999—"Long Term Care Insurance" By Robert J. Klosterman
The Sunday Capital, April 8, 2001—"Weighing the Cost of Long-term Insurance"

Chapter Eight

Washington Post, Sept 22, 2001,—"Traditional Houses Put Elderly at Risk"
AARP Bulletin, Sept 1993—"A Place to Call Your Own" By Leah K. Glasheen
Modern Maturity, May-June 1997—"NORC's: Staying Put and Happy" By Susan Levine
AARP Bulletin, Nov 1994—"My House is Your House" By Pat Shapiro
AARP Booklet—"Selecting Retirement Housing" D13680

Guide to Retirement Living—"Assisted Living Communities/Group Homes", "Options in Retirement Living", "Nursing Facilities"
AARP Bulletin, Feb 2000—"Looking for a place to live?"
USAA Magazine, Nov-Dec 1997, "A Toy Story"
The Capital—Family Living, "A few more suggestions for those who must grandparent from Afar" By Lois Wyse
Parade Magazine, March 16, 1997—"On Vacation With the Grandkids" By Joan Rattner Heilman
AARP Bulletin, Oct 1998—"Older Driving Safely" By William Barnhill
AARP Bulletin, Feb 1998—"You're in the driver's seat" By William Barnhill
Johns Hopkins Medical Letter, Sept 1999—"A Road Map for Staying Safe Behind the Wheel"
The Washington Post, April 20, 1997—"Fearless Traveler" By James T. Yenckel
MM, May-June 2001—"Snap Out of It: Best cures for jet lag" By Tom Dunkel
Southern Living—"Travel Tips For Overseas Flying"
Washington Post—"Selling Products for Seniors with a Flair" By Patricia Dana Rogers
Modern Maturity, Jan-Feb 2001—"Cool Aids" By Kathleen Doheny

Chapter Nine

Washington Post, May 13, 2003—"Dying on Your Terms" By Beth Baker
Bereavement Assistance Notes—"Planning for Present Peace of Mind" By Randy King
Washington Post/Health, April 20, 1999—"Where There's a Will" By Stan Hindon
Washington Post, Jan 16, 2000—"Handle the Estate With Care" By Albert B. Crenshaw

USAA Magazine, Jan-Feb 2000—"Could You Sell a Herd of Buffalo?" By Josie Corning
Retired Officer, July 2001—"At Ease" By Peter Weaver
Washington Post, April 10, 2000—"Added Grief for the Bereaved" By Caroline E. Mayer
Washington Post/Health, June 6, 2000—"For Organ Donation, a Kidney-Shaped Pool" By Don Colburn
Parade Magazine, Jan 5, 1997—"Discover Your Family History" By Jim & Terry Willard
AARP Bulletin, Jan 2002—""Preserving Wartime Memories" By Roberta Yared

LIST OF WEBSITES

AARP – Connections for Independent Living	*www.arrp.org/lsn*
Online retirement calculator	*www.aarp.org/bulletin*
Housing/ECHO	*www.aarp.org/echo*
Life Answers	*www.aarp.org/lifeanswers*
Grief and Loss	*www.aarp.org/griefandloss/*
Abledata	*www.abledata.com*
Accessible Journeys	*www.disabilitytravel.com*
Alternative Health News Online	*www.altmedicine.com*
Alternative Medicine Clearing House	*www.nccam.nih.gov*
Alzheimer's Association	*www.alz.org*
Alzheimer's Disease Education and Referral Center	*www.alzheimers.org*
American Academy of Anti-Aging Medicine	*www.WorldHealth.net*
American Academy of Audiology	*www.audiology.org*
American Association for Geriatric Psychiatry	*www.aagpgpa.org*
American Savings Education Council	*www.choosetosave.org*
American Board of Specialties	*www.certifieddoctor.org*
American Cancer Society	*www.cancer.org*
American Foundation for Suicide Prevention	*www.afsp.org*
American Heart Association	*www.americanheart.org*
American Institute for Cancer Research Nutrition Information	*www.aicr.org*
American Lung Association	*www.lungusa.org*
American Medical Association	*www.ama-assn.org*
American Sleep Apnea Association	*www.sleepapnea.org*
American Sleep Disorders Association	*www.asda.org*
Apple Systems	*www.apple.com/education/k12/disability*

Arthritis Foundation	www.arthritis.org
Assisted Living Federation of America	www.alfa.org
Association for Safe International Road Travel	www.asirt.org
Association of Cancer Online Resources, ACOR	www.acor.org
Automobile Association of America Foundation	www.aaafoundation.org
Baptist Bible College	www.bbc.edu
Capturing Memories	www.capturingmemories.com
Center for Mind Body Medicine	www.cmbm.org
Centers for Disease Control and Prevention	www.cdc.gov
Children of Aging Parents	www.caps4caregivers.org
Church of Jesus Christ Latter-Day Saints	www.familysearch.org
Consumer Product Safety Commission	www.cpsc.gov
Corporation for National and Community Service	www.seniorcorps.org
Cost Containment Research Institute	www.institute-dc.org
Doubleday Large Print Home Library	www.doubledaylargeprint.com
Earthwatch	www.earthwatch.org
Eastern Paralyzed Veterans Association	www.epva.org
Elder Care Online	www.ec-online.net
Elderhostel Service and Travel	www.elderhostel.org
Eqifax	www.equifax.com
Experian	www.experian.com
Family Tree Magazine	www.familytreemagazine.com
Federal Drug Administration	www.cfsan.fda.gov/~dms/foodlab.html
Footsmart Catalog	www.footsmart.com
Foundation for Grandparenting	www.grandparenting.org
Global Volunteers	www.globalvolunteers.org
Grandtravel	www.grandtrvl.com
Habitat for Humanity	www.habitat.org
Heart Information Network	www.heartinfo.org

Health Grades, Inc.	*www.healthgrades.com*
Holistic Medicine	*www.holisticmed.com*
Hospice Foundation	*www.hospicefoundation.org*
Identity Theft Resource Center	*www.idtheftcenter.org*
International Association for Medical Assistance to Travelers, IAMAT	*www.IAMAT.org*
Intervac International	*www.intervac.com*
Library of Congress – Talking books	*www.lcweb.loc.gov/nls*
American Folk Life Center	*www.loc.gov/folklife/vets*
Lighthouse for the Blind – Gold Violin Catalog	*www.goldviolin.com*
Mayo Clinic	*www.mayoclinic.com*
Education	*www.mayo.edu*
Medical Billing Advocates of America	*www.billadvocates.com*
Microsoft.com	*www.microsoft.com/enable*
Military Officer's Association of America	*www.moaa.org*
National Academy of Elder Law Attorneys, NAELA	*www.naela.com/naela/questions*
National Archives and Records Administration	*www.nara.gov*
National Arthritis & Musculoskeletal & Skin Diseases Information	*www.nih.gov/naims/*
National Association for Continence, NAFC	*www.nafc.org*
National Association of Professional Geriatric Care Managers	*www.caremanager.org*
National Cancer Institute	*www.cancer.gov*
Cancer Information Service	*www.nci.nih.gov*
National Council on the Aging	*www.benefitscheckup.org*
National Depressive and Manic Depressive Association	*www.ndma.org*
National Federation of the Blind	*www.nfb.org*
National Foundation for Alternative Medicine	*www.nfam.org*
National Institute on Aging	*www.nih.gov/nia*
National Institutes of Health – Medline	*www.nlm.nih.gov/medlineplus/ druginformation*

National Kidney & Urologic Diseases Information Clearinghouse.	www.nidik.nih.gov
National Mental Health Association	www.nmha.org
National Mobility Equipment Dealers Association	www.nmeda.org
National Rehabilitation Hospital Center for Health & Disability Research	www.nrhchdr.org
National Safe Kids Campaign	www.safekids.org
National Stroke Association	www.stroke.org
National Women's Health Resource Center	www.healthywomen.org
Neurology Information Office, NINDS	www.ninds.nih.gov
New York Times Large Type Weekly	www.nytimes.com
Office of Disease Prevention & Health Promotion	www.healthfinder.gov
Paralyzed Veterans of America	www.pva.org
Partnership for Caring	www.partnershipforcaring.org
Point of Choice	www.mealsforyou.com
Reader's Digest—Large Type	www.readersdigest.com
Rebuilding Together	www.rebuildingtogether.org
Sleepnet.com	www.sleepnet.com
Social Security	www.ssa.gov
	www.seniors.gov
Stanford University Medical Center's Health Library	www.healthlibrary.stanford.edu
TransUnion	www.tuc.com
Toy Manufacturers of America	www.toy-tma.com
Tufts University	www.navigator.tufts.edu
USDA Food and Nutrition Information Center	www.nal.usda.gov/fnic
US Department of Health and Human Services – Medicare	www.medicare.gov
Mental Health	www.hhs.gov
Organ donation	www.organdonor.gov
US Department of State – Bureau of Consular Affairs	www.travel.state.gov
Well Spouse Foundation	www.wellspouse.org
WGBH—Boston	www.wgbh.org

INDEX

A

AARP
  Fulfillment 51
Abuse 172
Acid Reflux Disease 71
Acupressure 120
Acupuncture 120
Advanced Directive 230
Albert, Marilyn, PhD 191
AlcoholBenefit of moderate
    amount 84
Alternative medicine 117
  Acupressure 120
  Acupuncture 120
  Aromatherapy 121
  Biofeedback 121
  Body/mind medicine 121
  Chiropractic Therapy 121
  Conventional Western 121
  Herbal 121
  Holistic 121
  Holistic treatment 120
  Homeopathy 122
  Naturopathy 122
  Osteopathy 122
  Practioners 43
  Safety 123
  Spiritual healing 122
  Therapeutic touch and massage 122
  used to treat depression 184
Alzheimers Disease 195, 211
  Caregiving 203
  Respite care 205
  Strategies 200, 203
  Symptoms 198
Amateur, Xavier Francisco 187
American Academy of Anti-aging
    Medicine 19
American College of Nutrition 45
American Dietetic Assoc 46
Anti-depressants 183
Aromatherapy 121

B

Baby Boomers 32
  Effect of aging 27

Bach, James F. and Phyllis 56
Baird, Pat 75
Baroudi, Carol. *See* John R. Levine
Beller, Susan Provost 311
Billig, Nathan, MD 22
Bipolar disorder 180, 182, 186
Blau, Sheldon P. 128
BMI Body Mass Index
   Formula for 65
Bodys needs changing 50
   Hair 52
   Hearing 54
   High blood pressure 55
   Kidney and bladder 52
   Osteoporosis 53
   Skin 55
   Taste and smell 54
   Teeth and gums 54
   Vision 53
Bratman, Steven 124
Breast cancer
   Risk assessment 114
Brookes, Tim 176, 305
Browning, Robert 38

C

Caregiving
   A checklist of questions 146
   Finding a nursing home 169
   Full service agency 161
   Knowing when to get involved 144
   Long distance 141, 167
   Partner as caregiver 164
   Shifting roles 149
Carlin, Vivian F. 255
Chiropractic threapy 121
Christianson, Stephen G. 299
Cognitive therapy 184
Cohen, Dr. Gene D. 204
Complementary medicine. *See*
   Alternative medicine

Condon, Gerald M. & Jeffrey L. 296
Constipation 74
Conventional western medicine 121
Croom, Emily 310
Crowe, Elizabeth Powell 311

D

Decluttering the house 288
Dementia 177, 192, 199
   Multi-Infarct 195
Depression 177
   Contagious 184
Depression,
   Poor nutrition, effects of 194
Dial a hearing screening test 54
Diarrhea 74
Dietician
   Description of 46
Digestive problems 70
   Acid Reflux Disease 71
   Constipation 73
   Diarrhea 74
   Gallbladder disorder 74
   Gluten intolerance 73
   Heartburn, acid reflux 71
   Irritable bowel syndrome 74
   Lactose intolerance 72
   Side effect of medicine 74
Disabilities
   Hearing Impaired 284
   Visually Impaired 285
Doctor/patient
   Office visits 104
   Relationships 103
Doctor/patient relationships
   Personal medical profile 107
Doctor/patient Second opinions 108
Doress-Worters, Paula B. 49
Driving
   Chiropractic therapy 121
   Driving safety 274

Finding other ways to get there 278
For the disabled 279
Giving it up 276
How accidents happen 273
Staying in the drivers seat 272
Ducasse, Elizabeth 157
Durable Health Care Power of
    Attorney 13
Durable Health Care Proxy 230, 233
Durable Health Power of Attorney 225
Durable Power of Attorney 230
Dychtwald, Ken 48

E

Eating well
    Evaluating studies 64
    Fats 61
    Lite 60
    Nutrition labels 60
    Red meat 59
    Serving size 58
    Sweeteners 63
Elder law service 219
Eldercare Locator 29, 169, 278
Electro-convulsive therapy 184
EMS Pallaiative Care/Do not
    resuscitate order 230
Estate Planning 220
Executor, being an 297
Exercise 66
    As treatment for depression 184
    Dealing with Arthritis 68
    Weight training 68

F

Financial planner 221, 222
Financial planning 221
    For aging parents 223
Friedan, Betty 26

Funeral 30
    Planning for 299
    Prepaid 302

G

Geriatric care manager 168
Geriatric specialist
    Description of 46
Gluten Intolerance 73
Golant, Susan K. 157
Goldberg, Burton 123
Gollobin, Charlotte 12
Gordon, Dr. James 117
Grandparents 264
    Family Friends Project 271
    Foster Grandparents 271
    Long distance grandparenting 269
    Safety for grandchildren 265
Grieving 304
Guardianship 230

H

Hannon, Kerry 212
Health care providers 11
    In the home 11
Health care proxy 230
Health Maintenance Organization,
    HMO 225
Heart disease 109
    Blood test results 110
Herbal medicine 44, 121
Holistic medicine 12, 121
Home health care
    Certified nursing assistant, CNA 154
    Companion/sitter 154
    Finding the best caregiver 155
    Gallbladder Disorder 74
    Geriatric care manager 155
    Homeopathy 121
    Hospice care 154

Intravenous therapy nurse 154
Licensed practical nurse, LPN 154
Registered nurse, RN 154
Respite care 155
Supervised adult day care 155
Visiting nurse 154
Home inventory 217
Hospice 11, 175, 290
Hospital
Avoiding mistakes 127
Being an advocate 129
Healing & recovery 140
Minimizing risk surgery 125
Nursing care after discharge 150
Serious or terminal illness 131
Housing options 242, 249
Alzheimers disease facilities 243
Assisted living 243, 248
Continuing or Lifetime Care 243
Continuing or Lifetime care 249
Downsize or renovate 242
Elder Cottage Housing Opportunity, ECHO 242, 253
Home renovation 244
Home share 247
Home-share 242
Moving in with the children 243, 253
Moving out/selling the house 251
NORC 246
Retirement communities 246
Safety considerations 245
Selling the house 242
Senior citizen residential communities 243

I

Identity theft 214
Credit report 215
Incapacity 11
Planning for 229

Integrative medicine. *See* Alternative medicine
Internet 13, 30
As research tool 262
Email 263
Evaluating information 100
Support groups, chat rooms 99, 102
Irritable Bowel Syndrome 74

J

Jamison, Kay Redfield 180
Josefowitz, Natasha 20

K

Kahn, Robert L. 21
Klein, Arthur C. *See* Dava Sobel 70

L

Lactose Intolerance 72
Lange. *See* Morris, Lois B
LeDoux, Denis 308
Letter of instruction 296
Levine, John R. 263
Light therapy 184
Living Will 13, 225, 230, 231
Long, Jane S & Richard W. 313
Long term health care insurance 226
waiver of premium 228
Lustbader, Wendy 165

M

Mace, Nancy L. 204
Manic Depressive illness. *See* Bipolar disorder
Mansberg, Ruth. *See* Vivian F. Carlin
Massage 122
McGowin, Diana Friel 199

McKhann, Guy, MD 191
Medicaid 225
Medical
  bills 135
  care planning 224
  personal profile 138
Medicare 205, 225, 231
Medicare HMO 225
Medicine
  Antacids 76
  Drug allergies 81
  Drug interaction 76
  Drug warning labels 82
  Laxatives 77
  Misuse 77, 79
  Non steroidal anti-inflammatory drugs 80
  Self diagnosis 76
Medigap insurance 225
Mediplus insurance. *See* Medigap insurance
Memories
  Family history/genealogies 309
  Leaving a legacy 306
  Professional papers/photographs 310
  Storing/protecting and preserving 312
  Writing a life story 307
Memory loss
  Evaluating 188
  Useful hints 190
Meyer, Marcia M. 166
Money managing 136
Morris, Lois B. 117
Morris, Virginia 146

N

National Center for Complementary and Alternative Medicine dicine 44

National Council on Aging
  Benefits check up 29
Naturopathy 121
Nesi, Thomas. *See* M. Michael Wolfe
Networking 237
Neuropsychiatry & Memory Clinic 192
Nutrition
  Key to good health 12
Nutritional therapy 184
Nutritionist
  Description of 45

O

Obituary writing 301
Organ donor 303
Orin, Rhonda 137
Ormond, Suze 212
Osteopathy 121

P

Patient Self-determination Act 231
Pelletier, Dr. Kenneth 47, 95
Personal information file 212
Pollin, Irene 157
Power of Attorney 229, 233
Prostate cancer 115
Provenance 296
Pseudodementia 193
Psychotherapy 184

R

Rabins, Dr. Peter V. 204
Reinhold, Arnold. *See* John R. Levine
Retirement
  Adjustment for spouses 35
  Financial planning 220
  Planning for 32

Possibilities 235
Right to die issue 232
Risen, Aura Epstein 187
Rosenfeld, Dr. Isadore 124
Rowe, Dr. John 21

S

Seasonal Affective Disorder, SAD 180
Settling the estate
    Clearing the family home 314
    Sharing the valuables 316
Sheehy, Gail 22, 38
Shenk, David 198
Shimberg, Elaine Fantle. *See* Blau, Sheldon P.
Siegal, Diana Laskin 49
Sleeping problems
    Insomnia 86
    Sleep apnea syndrome 90
Sobel, Dava 70
Social Security 29, 225
Sound partnership 209
Spiritual healing 122
Stanney, Barbara 42
Stroke, brain attack 111
Suicide 188
Support system 239

T

Therapeutic touch therapy 122
Totten Trust 302
Transitional, Acute care or Rehabilitation facility 152
Traveling
    Avoiding jet lag 282
    Medical care away from home 280
Tuttle, Craig A. 313

U

UC Berkeley Wellness Newsletter 51
Urinary incontinence 91
    Prostate problems 93

V

Vitamin and mineral deficiency 45

W

Wasserman, Selma 270
Weil, Andrew 119
Weil, Dr. Andrew 44
Western, allopathic medicine 117
Wills 292
    Personal gifts 295
    QTIP Trust 293
    Thinking of the grandchildren 294
Wolfe, M. Michael 75

Y

York, The Rev. Sarah 300
Young, Margaret Levine. *See* John R. Levine

NOTES

NOTES

Printed in the United States
82717LV00004B/117/A